A CLASS IN LIFE EXTENSION

A Primer for Extending your Life

BOB GUTH

Table of Contents

Revisions

This book is now in its fourth revision of the original text. This present 2022 edition is a total rewrite of the 2021 volume. I realized that the 2021 edition needed to have the material and practices and processes for longevity (or beginning life extension) reorganized into a separate and whole new section apart from the material for intermediate life extension, and so in this latest 2022 edition all of the more basic practices have been placed in their own section that I have called, 'Part 1, Beginning Practices of Life Extension.' And then continuing this theme, I reorganized all of the practices for intermediate life extension in its own section that I labeled, 'Part 2, Intermediate Practices of life extension.' And, of course, the last major section contains the more advanced practices and I have called it, 'Part 3, Advanced Practices for Life Extension.' And also, the affirmations have been separated and placed at the end of each of the three sections as they apply to each of the three sections. The material on breath work practices has been expanded to include the 'Breath of Fire', the 'Slow Breath' and the 'Precisely Timed Breath' and these all help to lead a life extension aspirant into the new human personality complex that begins to differentiate you as a life extender from the general population. I have consolidated the text and visualization-meditations for attaining a state of compassion and higher consciousness, and for avoiding the death hormone to make them easier to work with. Many of the visualization-meditations for life extension have been revised to add greater depth and make them more concise. Also, in many of them, I have added a line requesting you to bring in your spirit guide team to help you work with the guidance and benevolence that all of the interdimensional helpers can give us. Much new information, direction and guidance has been added to the advanced visualization-meditations. And I combined or moved a number of the more advanced life extension practices into different chapters or combined several of them into one chapter. And last, I decided to leave the number of chapters at 11 for a reason. And that reason is that 11 is a master number and it means master message. Perhaps this book with its 11 chapters can become a master message for you to help you extend your life.

Acknowledgements

I would like to express my gratitude and appreciation for the organizers of the annual RAAD Fest events. The RAAD Fest which began in 2016, and has continued every year since then is the major worldwide player in the new movement for life extension. Their focus is basically through using external science. RAAD stands for The Revolution Against Aging and Death (or Radical Life Extension), and the annual RAAD Fests have started a worldwide momentum for life extension. I am grateful for their work in putting together the annual RAAD Fest conferences that feature speakers from all over the world on anti-aging and age reversal technologies and breakthroughs. I am grateful to them because it was at one of those RAAD Fest events that I decided to start publishing my own writings on longevity and life extension, and this book is one of them. The RAAD Fest is a coalition of two organizations, People Unlimited, and the Life Extension Foundation. I also want to acknowledge the great help humanity has received from all of the higher dimensional beings who are speaking through human channels and who have been instrumental in helping to awaken the human race to a higher consciousness level of benevolence, kindness, brotherhood, peace, and especially the peaceful passing of the Dec 21, 2012 marker for the Armageddon. I also want to thank the many, many humans who are channeling this wisdom for higher spirituality and for life extension, and for the new technology; for their tireless work in bringing in this new information that has been revealed and is greatly needed. I also want to thank the higher dimensional beings for the dreams that were given to me on healing and longevity and life extension. I am sure that when you read some of these dreams you will also value their wisdom. I want to acknowledge and thank Dale Anderson for creating the pen and ink cover art drawing of students being taught by a master teacher near a Tibetan Monetary because his art work fits into the theme of this book so well. And I want to thank Jessica Guth, for her wonderful color rendering of Dale's cover art.

Prologue

What are some of the real causes of Aging? Why can't the body regenerate lost or damaged tissues? These are good questions and the answers will take us beyond conventional knowledge. Current theories on aging talk about DNA damage, the increase of senescence cells, mitochondria aging, free radical damage, telomere shortening, and others, but it is an ongoing research activity. I will list some of the other (real) causes of aging that have been revealed to humanity that you will read about in detail in this book. But it is important to know that there are also affirmations and meditations and energy exercises in this book that will help you avoid them. Your thoughts, beliefs and expectations about how long you think you can live are a big part of what causes aging. And this connects to what is called your death urges. Negative emotions, especially fear, create aging because fear opens up fissures in your auric field and this allows the fragmentation of a small part of your soul energy to fragment off and seep out depleting your life force energy and this causes aging. Another cause of aging is that your body has an aging clock which activates the death hormone release when people reach maturity at around age 35. This is an important and unrecognized reason why when people reach age 35, they start to age and decline. Toxins cause aging. Obvious toxins are the addictive substances, but there are many others including pesticide residues, chemicals and preservatives in foods and water. And also, there are hidden toxins such as the 150 parts per million of heavy water in all of the waters of the world and this causes aging. Major diseases wear the body down physically and the fear associated with them depletes life force energy and this is a part of aging. Diet plays a role. SAD [Standard American Diet] contributes to many diseases and does not supply enough energy for good body regeneration. And people have a negative bias from past and present life experiences that cause them to expect bad things to happen and this plays into the death urge and aging. Literature exists that says when a newborn first enters the world it senses the ambient energy and realizes that it is in a low energy environment and that there will only be enough energy available for body maintenance, but not enough to repair or regrow severely damaged or lost body parts or severely damaged tissues and structures, and this low energy level environment is part of the reason for sub-optimal human body regeneration. Humans have latent abilities that are dormant now, such as the 24th chromosome pair, and when this is activated, it can block disease and increase lifespan. Literature exists that says magnetic repolarization of the magnetic field of the DNA in the cells and organs of the body can allow humans to rejuvenate into longer life spans.

Introduction

In the 21st century the world has seen great changes and one of those is the idea that it is now becoming possible to extend your life. Indeed, the practices for immortality as taught by the ancient masters of physical immortality have become available in recent years. And many new spiritual technologies have been revealed to mankind to assist human longevity. In addition to this there are many new discoveries and inventions coming from external science to help humans live longer. Life extension is a fascinating subject, and one of the basic tenants that you will hear over and over again is that fundamentally, it is simply in the power of your mind. This one idea, "if you do not expect to age, you will not age," is at the heart of it. Easy to say, isn't it? And yet we all have a belief in aging. In this book, we will look at the fundamentals of reprograming your belief system which is the governor of your thought patterns, and it is your preponderant thought patterns that formulate (or reflect) to you, your body's external reality.

It is important to know that there are many, many practices, processes, and techniques, and technologies and that can extend your life. Your diet is one – the kinds of foods you eat and drink are a part of it. Keeping yourself in good physical condition, of course, is another. Not as well-known is the importance of maintaining a low risk profile for not getting any of the major diseases. Everyone knows that avoiding addictions plays a big role. But most people do not know that keeping your emotional state calm is indeed more important for your longevity than people realize. Taking better and better care of your physical body is part of the story too and not to be overlooked. Indeed, there are many, many things that play into this business of extending your life. However, the topics just mentioned are all third dimensional. It is a major mistake to think that longevity can only be found in the third dimensional realm.

What about higher dimensional aspects? Do you think that things that are higher dimensional can affect your longevity? Indeed, they can and there are many of them and in the not-so-distant future these higher aspects will be recognized as major players in life extension. The increasing lifespan among humans will be partly due to the greater knowledge and utilization of the higher dimensional aspects of the body. There are many, many factors that affect your lifespan that are not third dimensional, such as cleansing and shimmering your auric field, retrieving lost soul fragments, increasing your DNA efficiency, stopping your body's aging clock and death hormone releases, learning spiritual technologies, and of major importance, cultivating thoughts and emotions of a peaceful, contented, long-lived life extender.

The immortal masters of old always have taught the importance of cultivating the positive emotions of gratitude, compassion, and love because they know that negative emotions of the opposite kind such as resentment are important causes of aging. But there are many strictly third dimensional aspects that must be mastered too, such as earning a living, maintaining the proper weight, and moving to a longevity diet. Being overweight is a third dimensional important aging factor. Other causes of our current short life spans have to do with emotional aspects such as the aging toll caused by rampaging negative emotional outbursts. Another is the preponderant thought patterns of getting older by those who are getting older. And yet another is being overly serious and not letting your inner child out to play. It may surprise you to learn that (as of 2022) there are many people living now who are over 110. Wikipedia has articles listing the world's oldest men and women, and in 2022, there were a least 100 humans who were over 114! And the trend of people living longer is accelerating exponentially. In 1980 in the USA there were 32,000 people over 100, in 2010 there were 53,000, and there were 92,000 by 2020, and by 2060 it is projected that 600,000 people will be over 100 years of age. Leading scientists on aging all agree that either slowing our aging clock or even resetting it will be accomplished in the near future. In the future, life extension will become the new way of life and it is already starting. And rejuvenation is coming too. Some of the technologies for age-reversal that are currently being developed are: whole body stem cell makeover, young blood plasma, and CRISPR/Cas9 gene editing, and there are other anti-aging technologies being developed now and more advanced rejuvenation technologies will be developed in the future. There are forecasts that point to a 2045 timeframe when age-reversal and rejuvenation technologies will go mainstream.

One of the exciting reasons to begin the practices of life extension is to be here for rejuvenation. Yes, rejuvenation will be coming in the near future, and we will repeat it – there are futurists who predict that by 2045 age reversal technologies will be available. And there are already a number of new technologies that can revitalize, restore, and rejuvenate your body to some extent.

Part 1

Beginning Practices of Life Extension

CHAPTER 1
Traditional Immortality Practices

Life extension, can you see, is mostly in your mind, it's key
To a much longer life span – and is the future human legacy.
But enmeshed as we are in the mass consensus belief
In aging and death – we live and age and die in grief
With lives of struggle, stress and trouble without relief.
But if you can attain higher consciousness enough to know
That your life can flow on in ease and joy, then you can go
For life extension, and you can go for it even though
The masses lag behind until they too evolve enough to find
That they have just as much ability as anyone to be aligned
To the higher spectrum thoughts and emotions of the kind
That adores creation with life forms abounding all around –
And abhors war wanting world brotherhood to be found –
And sends compassionate action in ways that do astound!
If you can create thoughts and beliefs that allow you to relate
To life extension and if that way of life becomes what you create
Through your affirmations and life pattern changes then I'll state
That this indeed sets the stage for you to let your lifespan really soar
To at least 150 years and perhaps well past that for many years more!

It has been said that what you can do with the external sciences you can also do with the internal science, and that is indeed a true statement. There are legends of ancient immortal masters who lived 500 to 800 years in far east, in India and China, and they had no external technology. But they mastered the inner science, the internal technology, and that is how they were able to live so long. The ancient immortality aspirants (the students of the masters) were taught the traditional purification practices by the masters of the far east, and to the masters, one word said it all, and that one word was 'perfection.' But, the partner of perfection is 'purification,' and the ancient immortal masters developed techniques to condition and purify their minds such that they came to expect immortality. They worked daily to cultivate the mindset of an immortal master who was going to live 500 to 800 years. They used breathwork purification sessions to bring in vast amounts of oxygen and life force energy (prana) to add new energy to their bodies that in turn helped their bodies create new cells. And they used fasting purification to absorb and break down some of their body's old senescent cells and thereby stop the aging toxins that comes from those old cells. And they learned to work with and cultivate compassion, and they developed higher psychic abilities such as telepathy. And they evolved into ever higher levels of consciousness.

Recently a master was asked what could be done to help humans achieve longevity and life extension and the master said anything that has to do with bringing in more oxygen [and prana or life force energy]. Basically, life extension from the traditional practices involves developing a life extension mindset, then continually adding new energy (oxygen and parana) through breathwork to create new cells), then getting rid of old energy (dead or worn-out cells) by fasting, and then evolving into higher levels of consciousness. Listed below are some of the many practices of the inner science that the ancient masters of immortality used to attain their extreme longevity, their life extension.

Thought Purification – cultivating immortality thoughts and higher consciousness thoughts

Emotion Purification – cultivating higher spectrum emotions of compassion and love for all life

Death Urge Purification – Getting rid of the death urge and replacing it with the life urge

Breath Purification – breath work cycles, exhale expels toxins, inhale adds oxygen and prana

Fasting Purification – part of the masters and religious traditions for purification, purifies blood and flesh

Meditation Purification – cultivates calmness, even in the eye of a storm

Five Element Purification – earth (food), air (breath), water (drink), fire, aether

Bathing Purification – showers clean not only skin, but also removes aetheric toxins

Sleep and Gratification Purification – develops mastery over sleep and gratification

Community and Gaia Purification – develops deep relationship to community and Gaia

Mastery over the Physical Body – was central to the ability to attain immortality

The aspirant was taught many techniques and practices that demonstrated the mind's ability to control and master the body. Among them were fasting and breath mastery, meditation and commanding the body to absolute stillness.

Traditional Practices of Physical Immortality

Purification of Thoughts and Emotions

Students were tutored on the importance of training the mind and the emotions to create an immortal mindset. They were also taught the importance of choosing thoughts and emotions that were positive, helpful and for the good of all. And a great reverence for the gift of life was always taught. To honor and respect the rights of others to exist in happiness and joy was a discipline. Acolytes were tutored on training their emotions to be of a compassionate nature and to work on developing more love for everything around them, everything about them, and for themselves. They were taught to cultivate contentment no matter what their circumstances were. They were taught that all negative emotions create destructive energies that can wreak havoc on their own bodies and on their external world if they externalize their negative emotions. In the West, workshops on rebirthing and physical immortality focused upon saying physical immortality affirmations to reprogram the student's belief system which is the key to reprogramming their thought patterns for life extension. In the East, affirmations were also used to condition the minds of the students to accept the belief that the much longer lifespan of an immortal (one who could live three to five conventional lifespans) was possible for them. These affirmations were said over and over and over again so that they transitioned into an immortality mindset. They created the expectation for the students of the Taoists Masters in China and for some of Babaji's followers in India that they could live hundreds of years longer than was normal for the region. And now much new information has been revealed to humanity recently on life extension in years following 2012 that have added to the repertoire of practices for creating life extension. Life extension affirmations and the importance that thoughts and emotions have on life extension are covered in depth in later chapters.

Death Urge Riddance Purification

You will need to heal your death urge. Everyone has a death urge. It is a culturally cultivated reaction to stress, harshness, disappointment, feeling left out, feeling unwanted, and feeling frustration. The death urge is a big cause of death. The reality is that most people who succumb to their death urge and will themselves to die could actually have lived much longer. And people who are enmeshed in their death urge tend to have a belief that it is normal to die at 60 to 80 because, they will tell you, that is what people do. This needs to be looked at and healed because it is this belief in and of itself that will limit you in your potential longevity. The opposite is really true – you have the potential to reach your natural life span of 140 to 150 years if among other things you can heal your death urge.

You must firmly state that you do not want to die – you want to live! It is important for the life extender to pull themselves out of this death urge business. Life is for living. Life is for loving. Life is for experiencing the new. Life is for enjoying all of the great changes that are all about us. Life is for seeing the age of humans maturing. Life is for being around to see the eventual coming together of all of the peoples of the world as a whole unified world population. Life is for looking at more and more people

putting aside the old ways of separation and war and evolving into the new paradigm of integration and cooperation into eventually, a unified world. This is highly exciting, is it not! This is not a death urge. This is a life urge.

Let the great gift of life deeply seep into you, deeply seep, seep like it is the tea of life. Why would you want to leave? It is important to reorient your thought streams into the creative aspects of the life extender. It is important to do the things you really enjoy doing. It is good to add new things that give you joy. Perhaps go to an opera, or a movie, or try a symphony, or a concert. Visit museums, go on retreats, attend workshops, develop new skills, create a business, get involved with community and civic and political groups working to bring about improvements. Become an inventor. Write books. Create works of art. Write songs, music and poetry. Become socially active. Develop stimulating relationships. Become an expert on one or more subjects. Take those vacations you've always wanted to take. In short enjoy life.

Make life fun. Make life interesting. Make life challenging. Make life a continual learning experience. Learn to enjoy learning new things just like a child does. Learn to enjoy music and its composition subtleties. Learn to enjoy dance and the uniqueness of the dance movement. Learn to enjoy how those great artists developed their creative talents. Ask to have some of their skills downloaded into your own consciousness. Make an intention to become your own genius self. Say the words, "I am becoming a genius, I am becoming a genius, I am becoming a genius," over and over. Study the lives of the great creators of the past and present – Mozart, Picasso, Tolkien, Dostoyevsky. Why would you want to leave early? It is simply a matter of saying, "Well, I had a bad time here or a bad month there, but all of that will pass, and I'm not going to let it dampen my enthusiasm for living. For life is what I'm all about. I want to live! I want none of this death urge stuff in me. I choose to get rid of all of my death urge impulses and replace them with my life urge impulses to experience the joy of life. I choose to let my life urge creative expressions flourish. I choose to get them out into the world because they are needed, and I am the only one who is going to be able to do it. So, go away, death urge. I have no time for you. My time is devoted to the thousand and one creative projects that I need to accomplish in my very, very long, life time." And that is all there is to it! And so, it shall be!

Breathwork Purification

Breathing techniques were so important to the eastern yoga masters that special terms were developed to allow for a sharper focus and a clearer understand of the various breath cycles and breathing techniques that were part of their daily lives. Chief among them were the many pranayama breath practices in which great amounts of oxygen and prana (or life force energy) were taken in with the inhale, and toxins were expelled through the exhale. In the west, conscious-connected breathing techniques were taught in rebirthing and physical immortality workshops. But many other breathwork practices exist, and the Breath of Fire is one of them. Also, a precisely timed breath cycle exists in which the in-breath and the out-breath are controlled to the thousandths of a second, and this helps to develop mastery of the mind over the body. Another is the very slow breath rhythm that can be used to calm and an anxious mind and control erratic emotions. All of these practices are important, and they oxygenate the entire system and bring in vast amounts of prana or life force energy (which is mixed in with the air) and this enlivens and rejuvenates the entire body. We should note that there are many other breathwork practices that exist that we won't have space to cover, but they can be found in literature on breathing practices.

In yogic traditions, the in-breath is the movement and activity of spirit, and the out-breath is the movement of air. In these traditions, breathwork sessions are continued until spirit (the source of breath) is merged with the air. When understood and mastered this is a direct and practical way of merging spirit and air right inside the human body. Yoga masters also teach their students that the body is fueled to the greater extent by the oxygen and prana life force energy that is taken in through the breath and the chakras, and it is fueled to a lesser extent by the food and drink that is consumed. Breath work sessions can also remove deep-seated trauma if the intention to do this is stated as a goal before the breathwork session begins. Indeed, it is very important to release deep-seated trauma because if left in the body these karmic elements will tend to block your personal transformation. Ideally, the breath should be taken in through the nostrils and not the mouth, because when the air comes in through the nostrils, it puts a spin on the air and this spin adds more energy to the air and when it enters the blood stream it brings more energy to the blood and this creates a bright red oxygenated blood that energizes the whole body. But if the nostrils are plugged, mouth breathing is all right.

Breath mastery techniques are powerful practices for life extension. These breath mastery practices will bring in vast amounts of oxygen and prana and the life extension student should make an intention both before starting and after completing a breathwork session that this extra oxygen and prana are to be used for body healing, repair and regeneration. You should speak out loud in a low voice before and after each breathwork session and say that you want the extra oxygen and prana to energize, repair, regenerate and youth your physical body.

The Breath of Fire

In rebirth and physical immortality workshops the conscious connected breathing rhythms were taught. Conscious Connected Breathing is simply breathing at a more rapid pace or cycle than the normal breathing rhythm. The sessions can be any length, but typically they are 5 to 15 minutes. There are many variations on the speed of the exhale-inhale cycle, but it is always faster than normal. Hour long Conscious Connected Breathwork sessions surprisingly enough have the power to heal deeply buried emotional traumas when that is stated as a goal before the session begins, and if this happens the rebirth-breather will feel a painful deeply buried emotional trauma come up to the surface and then start to cry, which allows them to release that trauma and this frees up the space it was taking making available more room for life force energy. The Breath of Fire technique is very similar to Conscious Connected Breathing but, in the Breath of Fire, the inhale is passive and the exhale is forceful. The exhale, requires contracting the abdominal muscles with the diaphragm, and this creates a noticeable in-out abdominal motion, and the diaphragm visibly moves back and forth during the inhale-exhale. The inhale and exhale should be the same length, with no pauses in between. The breaths are short and fast. The movement might be considered similar to panting.

Start with the exhale, then rapidly inhale-exhale, inhale-exhale, inhale-exhale at a faster than normal pace, short but fast breaths, moving large volumes of air and prana into and out of the lungs. Exhale at a faster than normal pace, then inhale at a faster than normal pace in a continuous rhythm. In rebirthing sessions this Conscious Connected Breathing is continued for an hour, but in daily breathwork sessions, two or three sessions, each lasting 3 to 5 minutes, is enough. The Breath of Fire is very similar to conscious connected breathing and basically replaces it. For the Breath of Fire, add the rapid forceful exhale by pushing your diaphragm in with your abdominal muscles, then passively inhale using your diaphragm. Move your diaphragm back and forth during each inhale-exhale cycle. Continue the Breath of Fire for two or three sessions, with each session lasting 3 to 5 minutes or you can go for one 15-minute session.

Pranayama Breathwork

This is a fundamental practice of the ancient immortals and there are many variations to this and special terms are often used, but the basic practices are quite straightforward and easy to understand. Called Kumbhaka Pranayama, there is a holding pattern at the end of each inhale and exhale. This offers the great advantage of bringing in much oxygen and prana life force energy and the holding of the breath after the exhale forces the brain and body to search for more oxygen. The holding of the breath at the end of the inhale drives this extra oxygen into the bloodstream and saturates the brain and body with oxygen, and it drives the extra prana into the energy meridian system. In doing this, it can become a very powerful tool for triggering ongoing body cellular regeneration for life extension and youthing. In the eastern traditions, yogi breath masters would have their students sit in a comfortable position on a mat, on a chair, or for the advanced, in the lotus posture. Then they would ask their adepts to calm themselves to stillness and focus on their breathing, on the in-breath and on the out-breath. Then instructor would then guide them in one of the many pranayama breathing rhythms. In pranayama breathing there are a thousand variations to the hold pattern. Some start with a mild hold pattern using a hold count of 4, (1001, 1002, 1003, 1004) for five to twenty breath rounds, holding the exhale and inhale at this count after each exhale and inhale. Then they might increase the hold count, to a count of 5 for another session of breath rounds. Then they might increase it again to 6, then 7, and then on to an 8-count hold for a full pranayama breathwork session. Masters go to even longer hold counts of 10, 11, and 12. Of course, the number of rounds for each hold count can vary too. This is a very powerful way to bring great amounts of oxygen and prana energy into your body. It is good to feel as if your brain and body become saturated with oxygen and prana energy during the inhale hold. Before and after each breathwork session state that you want this extra oxygen and prana to repair, regenerate and youth your body for life extension.

Speak out loud in a low voice and say that you want this extra oxygen and energy used to repair, regenerate and rejuvenate you for life extension.

Start with the exhale, slowly and completely empty the lungs to a count of 4, (one thousand one, one thousand two, one thousand three, one thousand four). Then hold with the lungs completely empty to a count of 4. Then quickly inhale, completely filling the lungs, and then hold with the lungs completely full to a count of 4. Do several rounds of this, perhaps six. Then continue with the 5-count hold for six rounds. Then repeat with a 6-count hold and continue with the 6-count hold for six rounds. Then repeat this cycle with an increased 7-count hold. Then repeat with a hold count of 8, and then 9. Continue this for 3 – 5 minutes or you can go for a 15-minute session.

Precisely Timed Breathwork

This technique is very useful for developing body mastery and it can also bring about body purification and cleansing. The precise timing of the inbreath-outbreath cycle in which each inhale and exhale are of the same duration, not varying by more than a hundredth of a second, demands and helps to develop concentration. Body purification comes about when one visualizes toxins and degenerated, worn-out tissues, as black specks being pulled out, and streaming out of the body with the air with each exhale. And then on each inhalation, prana is visualized as streaming in through all of body's major and minor spinning chakra energy vortexes. With each inhale visualize your body as an interdimensional body and see in your visualization prana energy streaming in through all of your 7 major chakras: the root, the navel, the solar plexus, the heart, the throat, the third eye, and the crown; and then visualize prana flowing into through all of your 114 minor chakras, at the bottoms of your feet, on your ankles, behind your knees, behind your shoulders, on your palms, wrists, elbows, behind your head, and many other locations and see this energy flowing into your 7200 nadis or energy meridian lines. This helps to develop mastery over your body. This breath technique requires neither deep breathing nor rapid breathing. Visualize your body as an interdimensional energy system and visualize that it has major and minor chakras and a vast meridian energy system in which energy is constantly flowing. Make an intention before starting and after completing this breathwork that the added oxygen and prana and the expelled toxins are all used for body healing, repair, and regeneration to extend your life.

Begin by concentrating on your breathing and bring it to your normal breathing cadence. Then begin to focus on the timing of each inhale and each exhale and intend to make them the same. Develop a timing rhythm cadence that is exactly the same length for each exhale and each inhale to a hundredth of *a second to best of your ability. After you develop a comfortable exact timed rhythm, begin to bring in the visualization of toxins streaming out with each exhale and prana streaming in through the breath and through all of the open chakras with each inhale. Begin to visualize your chakras as spinning vortexes of energy in all of your major and minor chakras starting at the bottoms of the feet, at the ankles, behind the knees, solar plexus, the hearth, in front of and behind the spine, the back of the shoulders, the throat, the third eye, the crown, and behind the head. Visualize prana streaming in through them and toxins with each inhale, and toxins and dead tissue streaming out with the exhale. Continue for 3 - 5 minutes or one 15-minute session*

The Slow Calming Breath

A very slow breathing rhythm can be useful for controlling stress and anxiety. During states of high anxiety both the heartbeat and breath rate increase dramatically and erratically and when the breath is purposely brought back to a very slow inbreath-outbreath rhythm it can control and coax the heartbeat into calmness and peacefulness.

Begin by bringing the breath to a very slow rate and after a few minutes notice how your heart beat has slowed to match your breathing and notice how this brings you back into a state of calmness and peacefulness. Continue until a state of peacefulness is reached.

My Breathwork Sessions

Here is a breathwork session I do. I combine these four breathwork techniques in the following order: Breath of Fire, Pranayama, Precisely Timed, and the Slow Breath. The number of exhale-inhale breath cycles in each varies but it is in the 2-to-5-minute range for each of the breath types: Breath of Fire, Pranayama, Precisely Timed; but for the Slow Breath it is perhaps just one minute to feel the calmness that it brings. One cycle of my breathwork session will include all four the breathwork types.

I do three cycles in a breathwork session. Three cycles of all four breaths at one breathwork session takes around 15 to 20 minutes. During the Pranayama sessions, I vary the hold pattern such that I may start the first inhale-exhale round with a 5-count hold, then increase it in the second round to a 6-count, then up it a 7, 8 and 9 hold count. During the last pranayama cycle of my breathwork session I may go for longer hold counts of 10, 11, 12 like the masters do. During the Precisely Timed Breath, I visualize myself as an interdimensional being and I visualize all of my major and minor chakras as energy vortexes and I visualize prana energy flowing into them during each inhale. On each exhale, I visualize worn out cells and toxins being pulled out and then streaming out with the air. I choose early morning right after I say my daily morning affirmations to do my daily breathwork session partly because air pollution is lowest at that time. And before I start my daily breathwork session I say out loud in a low voice, "I request and intend that the extra oxygen and prana energy from my breathwork session be used to repair my body, initiate regeneration, allow youthing, and create life extension."

My Breathwork Session
One cycle consists of doing all four breath types
I Repeat each cycle of the four breaths three times
Breath of Fire – 2-3 minutes
Pranayama – 2-3 minutes
Precisely Timed – 2-3 minutes
Slow Breath – 1 minute

Note also that there is a long list of curing the so-called incurable diseases through the major breath work practices. Large amounts of toxins can be expelled through the breath. Trauma can be released through breathwork. The body can be fueled through breathwork. Breathwork practices can purify the blood. Is it any wonder that pranayama breathing and other breathwork practices were a major part of the purification practices of the ancient yoga masters of immortality?

Fasting Purification Mastery

Fasting has always been a prime and important major body purification practice that the masters of physical immortality religiously used in all traditions of physical immortality. Fasting has always been a practice taught by the ancient master of immortality in the Taoist communities of China and by Babaji of India. Indeed, the notion of fasting for purification is steeped in religious traditions and many religions have fasting rituals. The 1-day a week fast is taught to beginning aspirants by Babiji. This is continued for 1-year to allow it to become an established life pattern habit. And then aspirants are asked to extend the fast to 3-days a week, again for a period of 1-year to adjust the body's rhythm to this purification. After that longer and more extended fasts are mastered. For the past 30 years I have been fasting 1-day a week, usually on Mondays, because I have fewer social obligations on that day. A fast of 1-day a week improves digestion and elimination. It helps to controls weight, makes food taste better after the fast, and it increases your ability to develop the strong willpower that it takes to do this. It does take willpower. When you fast 1-day a week you are going against your culture's eating conventions. You will be doing something that almost no one else will do or even consider doing. But I am not a fanatic about fasting either. Like everything, it is good to take a break from it once in a while. I do not fast when I am on vacation, mostly because part of the joy of a vacation is to eat the local foods where you are. But on Monday, I usually fast, I actually prefer it. Many longevity experts recommend fasting at least 1-day a week. It is a good idea to read up on fasting.

Intermittent Fasting has become popular in recent years and some may want to start with it. It should be mentioned also that medical science has discovered in their studies that old senescence cells in the body that accumulate with age release a cascade of toxins that cause aging, and some of these old cells can be removed through fasting. Fasting is covered in depth in later chapters, and it is covered extensively in chapter 11.

Purification Through Meditation and Stillness

Meditation is another important part of the practices taught that were taught to trainees in the immortality schools of the Taoists and by Babaji, and I have heard of several case histories in which severely traumatized individuals that were on a downward health spiral and were totally unable to function were completely cured through lengthy meditation. This, of course, is unconventional but the results can be remarkable. In one case of note, a client was instructed to simply meditate for perhaps one hour a day every day. And in the meditation the client was instructed to go to their place of perfect peace, or perhaps the great void. In either case they were to feel that there is no space, no time, no thought, no emotion, no worry, only peace, nothing but peace and themselves in their place of perfect peace or the great void and to just be there. The clients were instructed to allow no trauma to enter their meditation. All trauma (emotional or from injuries) was to be left behind. Usually this was very hard at first, but little by little, when they got used to the routine it became easier and easier, and slowly but surely, bit by bit, they began to recover and heal as their mind and their thoughts and emotions became more and more attuned to peace and calmness, and their physiological systems became more and more normally balanced. This shows plainly that the body has enormous capacity for healing and restoring itself back into a balanced state of perfect wholeness and health when all of the emotional trauma is released. When all of the body's systems, and parts and functions work together as an integrated wholeness team, then the body is healed. It also shows that many people create their own plunge into illness in the first place, due to a shock trauma, or from suffering a major injury. Meditation, in which thought-power has also been used to knit back and heal severely damaged tissue, bones, and organs and has also achieved very impressive cures that had been labeled as totally impossible cases beyond all hope.

Indeed, meditation is a very powerful and important practice. The calming affect that comes from meditation is very helpful for the life extender. It is a mark of mastery to develop the ability to maintain the physical form in a continual state of equanimity, peacefulness and contentment and in a sort of reverence for life. Yes, and even to have compassion for those who have a more negative agenda, for in the state that mediation can bring, you begin to realize that it is only through the life circumstances that those who work in negative ways choose that path. Indeed, it would be very good to read literature on meditation and then begin to add it to your daily life.

One of the easiest things you can do to help create and maintain thought patterns of a life extender is to practice the art of stillness. This is because being able to command your body to become perfectly still to the point where you could be mistaken for a statue is of great value because it will give you evidence that you can command your body to follow what your mind dictates. In this case, simply proving to yourself that you can become as still as a statue, not even blinking an eye, simply because your mind dictates it, is one small step to mastery. Eventually, over time, this will play into your belief system. If you can command your body to absolute stillness, then you can also command your body to extend your life span.

Pick any comfortable meditation position you choose. Command your body to go into perfect stillness such that the only moving thing in your body is your lungs and they are moving in a very slow, precise inhale and exhale breathing rhythm. Keep this up and practice keeping your body perfectly still for three to five minutes.

Purification with the Five Elements

Traditionally students were taught purification by working with the earth, air, water, fire and the aether elements. The earth element relates to food and drink. Aspirants were taught the basics of purer foods and drink. Recommendations for diets of food and drink for longevity and life extension were made. Consuming mostly organic vegetables, fruits, raw eggs, raw unpasteurized dairy, unsalted, unroasted nuts and seeds, and cooked starches and legumes (beans and peas) was encouraged with the idea of eventually becoming a vegetarian. Learning to eat less and to apply the energy formerly used for digestion and assimilation for elevating your consciousness was suggested. Learning to bless the food that you eat as well as the manner in which you eat it was honored. The water element relates to bathing in water to purify the body. The air element relates to breath work. The fire element relates to healing or transmuting negative emotions, and indeed, being near a fire has a very transmuting effect on the emotions. It is a good idea to sit by a fire just as the ancients used to do once in a while – it will transmute negative energy and restore calmness and peace even in our own rush-rush world. Purification with the aether involved smudging with smoke to remove negative energy in a space that had been used by others.

Purification Through Bathing

Some of the ancient eastern masters in India recommended bathing in the Ganges River twice a day, once in the morning and again in the evening. However, these days those river waters in India are too polluted and it's not such a good idea anymore. Yet the idea behind it is correct for several reasons. First, when one cleanses the physical body through a shower, the act of cleansing the body tends to spill over into the idea of cleansing the mental and emotional bodies from the spectrum of negative thoughts and emotions that may be there. Second, the body picks up not only physical toxins from the foods you eat and drink and the air you breathe, but it also picks up the aetheric components of these toxins. These aetheric toxins can be removed by a stream of fresh water running over your skin, and in fact your body places these aetheric toxins just outside your skin for this very purpose. That is why after you shower, you sometimes feel surprisingly deeply cleansed because the aetheric toxins have been washed away.

Mastery Over Sleep and Gratification

There were other areas of mastery that that aspirants were also taught and encouraged to master. They included learning to go without sleep and controlling the gratification urges. Some the masters could sit in meditation for days, weeks, or even months without sleeping.

Cultivating Community and Working with Gaia

The students were also taught the importance of belonging to community. They were coached to get involved with community and to bring harmony and higher spiritual values to the community and to work for improvements to eliminate some of the current difficulties. And always they were always taught to respect and honor and care for and work with the earth mother, Gaia, and all of the creatures that live upon her.

Developing Mastery

Humans tends to like to do things with others. It is a way of validating yourself through the seeming approval and acceptance of others who are doing the same thing such as exercising in a fitness club with many others. This desire for validation could be called the human standard. But a master does not need that sort of connection or validation from the others. A master is able to do what he or she knows is good for their body on their own. A master can do what he or she needs to do to create life extension on their own. It is a good idea to develop some of these traits of the masters.

Perfection in the Traditional Practices means Mastery of the Mind over the Body

CHAPTER 2
Modern Life Extension Practices

The technologies for age reversal and rejuvenation are now a major focus of hi-tech medical science and a large number of new startups have come into existence to develop life extension and age reversal technologies. The momentum for discovering age reversal technologies is on an exponential upswing. Starting around 2016, it has been accelerating faster every year. As of 2022 there are at least three medical science approaches for age-reversal and rejuvenation: whole body stem cell makeover, replacing old blood with new blood plasma, and a gene editing procedure called CRISPR. Futurists predict that these technologies and many others for age reversal will go mainstream by 2045. However, these technologies as of 2022 are in the early developmental stage, they are not completely proven, they have not undergone rigorous testing, and even if available they are prohibitively costly. It is likely that it will be two or three decades before they can receive regulatory approval and appear at an affordable cost. For the present, in 2022, it is important to look at the many other considerations and aspects that play into the modern approach to life extension. And one of the most important of these is to learn how to be able to live your life without fearing disease. You will need to learn how to live without fearing you could get some terrible life-threatening disease. It is necessary to also look at food choices you can make for extending your life, and the foods you should avoid that can be harmful and even shorten your life. And of course, we cannot overlook addictions that will rob you of many years. It is important to look at keeping your body physically fit and flexible, and to take better and better care of your body, and to provide for all your life's needs and expenses.

Thoughts and Emotions

There are a large number of new revelations for life extension that have been revealed to humanity. These revelations for life extension are quite numerous and are very, very important and need to made available to all who are drawn to want to live longer and extend their lives. And they were given in such a way that they can be easily understood and worked with so that they can be incorporated and integrated into the consciousness of the life extension student. Chapter 6, in its entirety is devoted to re-programming your thoughts, beliefs and emotions towards attaining life extension.

Learning How to Live Without Fearing Disease

One of the most important things you will need to learn is how to go forward in life without fearing that you might get some terrible life-threatening disease. This may sound difficult, but I don't think it is hard to do. I don't worry about getting any of the major diseases and I don't think it would be difficult for anyone else to learn how to not worry about it either. Basically, it has to do with maintaining a very low risk profile for not getting any of those serious diseases and illnesses. What may be surprising is that this goes far beyond just looking at the physical aspects of disease. It goes into acknowledging the ability of your mind and your emotions to actually create disease. It has been said that thoughts from the mind are basically used by all humans in a negative way at this time. Your mind can and does predisposition you to attract many of the diseases you fear. In order to develop the ability to live without fearing disease you will need to learn to direct your mental thought processes into states where you always choose to not focus on or worry about any disease. Instead, you will create preponderant thought patterns of maintaining your health. Your emotions also have a powerful effect in creating disease. The stronger you fear some disease and the more you worry about it, the more emotive power you put into energizing your fearful worrisome thoughts about it. And because of the power of the Universal Law of Thought, any great emotional out-pouring over any disease will create its manifestation that much faster, and then it will become that much more difficult to bring the body back into balance and health.

Preventing and Curing Heart Disease

Preventing heart disease on the physical level involves avoiding cooked fat foods that cause plaque in the arteries, not smoking or drinking alcohol, maintaining your correct body weight, exercising regularly and keeping your stress level low. On the mental side it will have to do with stopping a predilection to put yourself in positions of needing to accomplish overwhelming tasks that put you under great stress and time pressure. On the emotional plane it requires learning to be slow to anger and learning to maintain calmness under demands and pressures. Routine exercise and meditation contribute to prevention and healing. Also, there is the symbolism of heart disease. What is the symbol of the heart? The heart is the symbol of love on Valentine's Day cards. Symbolically, heart disease is a lack of self-love that happens when one is driven to accomplish some goal that is very difficult regardless of the toll it takes. The cure for heart disease may require a change in life style along the lines of what will prevent it. Also, choosing a diet for life extension substantially reduces the risk. And if you are told that you have plaque buildup in your arteries, there are ways of removing it, and colon hydrotherapy is said to be one of them.

Preventing and Curing Cancer

Cancer cures on the dietary level are well documented in the books of dietary healers, notably those of Vonderplanitz and others who prescribe the basic raw food diet which consists of raw dairy (unpasteurized milk, cream, cheese and butter), fresh organic vegetable juice, fresh organic fruits, uncooked eggs, unheated honey, cooked starches and legumes, and unsalted, un-roasted nuts and seeds. Routine exercise and meditation also contribute to prevention and healing. Often an emotional shock trauma is involved as explained in Dr. Rike Hamer's, New Medicine. A shock trauma might be getting a divorce, getting fired, getting a life-threatening disease, or becoming homeless. These must be acknowledged, worked with, remedied, and forgiven emotionally and mentally. Symbolically the rapid proliferation of cancer cells in a tumor represents the body's attempt to cope with a life-threatening situation – it may be a life shock (such as a divorce) or it may be an unlearned soul lesson (such as trying to control others). Curing cancer requires an extended period of cleansing with the basic raw food diet, and then integrating the shock trauma with forgiveness and by learning the soul life lesson involved. Adopting a healthier diet than the Standard American Diet (SAD) similar to the Mediterranean Diet, or better, a real, life extension diet, such as the Primal Diet of Vonderplantiz, will also help to prevent it. Cutting back on eating meat which has a 30% higher cancer risk is helpful. And a new product called Lite Water is said to gives an extra prevention boost and even a cure when it is injected into a tumor. And in the future, it is predicted that it will be discovered that an energy beam from the inert gas argon will be useful in disrupting an interdimentional aspect of this disease.

Preventing and Curing Diabetes

Diabetes is on the rise worldwide especially in developed countries and it is basically associated with being overweight, consuming sugar laden processed foods and drink, and living a life that lacks sweetness. Routine exercise and reversing an overweight condition are very helpful and often reverse it. Adopting a better diet (especially a diet for life extension) and avoiding all foods containing processed sugar is a big step towards curing it. Symbolically, the breakdown of the pancreas (or the inability of the gland responsible for utilizing that which is sweet in foodstuffs) points to (symbolizes) an imbalance in the life of the diabetic in which there is typically a lack of sweetness in the incarnation in progress. Many overweight diabetics do not enjoy the sweetness of experiencing sexuality and so the symbol is plain – the diabetic's body becomes unable to utilize sweet sugar nutrients which is directly symbolic of the diabetic's unwillingness to allow the sweetness of sexuality or other sweet life experiences into their reality. It is easily prevented by avoiding processed sugar foods, maintaining the proper weight, adopting a better diet than the Standard American Diet, exercising, meditating, and allowing a sweeter life style.

Preventing Dementia

This disease is another worry for older people and it is causes fear because orthodox medicine has no cure for it at this time. However, a study showed marked improvement in subjects who were put on and stayed on a routine exercise program. Dementia basically has to do with over mentalizing, being grumpy, unhappy, chronically angry, and harboring strong emotional feelings of not getting much out of live for the effort they feel they put into it. Adopting a raw food diet (especially raw dairy) is helpful and treatments such as hyperbaric oxygen and colloidal silver may show some reversal. Symbolically, this affliction represents the sufferer leaning too much towards the mental side of the three-sided triangle of beingness: the physical, the emotional, and the mental. So, the location of this affliction in the mind symbolically gives a message to the suffers subconscious that he or she has become out of balance especially in not allowing the positive emotions to flourish and not allowing the body to experience the joy of physical expression. The prevention of this disease is to exercise, eat a healthier diet, and to allow the emotional and physical sides of the triangle of beingness their expression of contentment, happiness, creativity, pleasure and body health. All of these need to be allowed to bloom. Also, there are some testimonials suggesting that radon spas and radon health mines are helpful.

Preventing and Curing Other Diseases

Other diseases such as pneumonia, emphysema, diarrhea, MERSA, kidney and liver disease, and a viral pandemic like COVID-19 can be prevented, and cured or controlled. Pneumonia, diarrhea and MERSA are inflammatory infectious bacterial diseases and so the prevention and cure for them will always involve keeping yourself healthy and physical fit in the first place, and then using a broad spectrum anti-microbial product. Colloidal silver is an effective broad spectrum anti-pathogen water solution of silver ions. Many testimonials exist on the effectiveness of colloidal silver in treating bacteria and virus-based diseases. Traditional medicine has many effective antibiotic drugs also. Emphysema, of course, has to do with smoking, and its prevention and cure are obvious. Kidney and liver disease are related to poor diet, and addictions that damage the body's filtering functions through the consumption of poisonous toxins (tobacco, alcohol and opiates), and also from indulging in toxic thoughts and emotions. Preventing and healing these afflictions requires the sufferer to stop the addiction and stop consuming the poisonous toxins, and then to stop the propensity for indulging in hateful toxic thoughts, and in chronically indulging in emotional upheavals from the whole range of negative emotions. Healing these negative emotional traits will require deep, deep healing. Surviving a pandemic, such as COVID-19, requires keeping yourself reasonably healthy and physically fit in the first place, and then using a broad spectrum anti-microbial substance such as colloidal silver to treat your symptoms if they become serious or difficult. Heat treatments from a hot soak also reduces symptoms, and inhaling Brown's Gas dramatically reduces inflammation in the lungs. And orthodox medical treatments for COVID-19 are important for life threatening cases.

What else can you do?

There are many other things you can do and they include basic physical, emotional, mental, nutritional and financial health. Fundamentally, you will need to keep yourself physically healthy. This means you will need to maintain a healthy life style and keep physical fit through regular activities that include fitness and flexibility exercise. Why is that? Because a healthy body fights off disease much better than an unhealthy body or sickly body does. Exercise is important but it is important to not overdo it and live in a fitness center. It is also important to eat a more healing and nutritionally supportive diet, and avoid getting enmeshed in the mass fear phobia of disease because all thought creates.

Learn to See All Disease as a Cleansing Opportunity

There is actually a much higher understanding about disease that needs to be made known. All microbial infections, actually all diseases, offer a cleansing opportunity. Why is that? Because in the case of infectious diseases, the microbial agents break down tissues better and faster than anything else can. Anyone with this higher knowledge about this positive cleansing aspect of a bacterial or viral infection knows that after it has run its course they will feel better afterwards because some of the deep-seated toxins will have been removed. And any microbial infection will run its course if it is in a human body that is kept healthy, gets enough exercise, consumes a nutritional healing diet, and maintains healthy emotions and beneficial mental thought patterns. This applies to an even difficult virus infections such as the COVID-19 virus that the world had never seen before, and therefore and had not developed any immunity to it. Anyone who has this higher knowledge, this higher wisdom, would not fear the coronavirus or any other similar infection! This higher knowledge, that all disease offers a cleansing opportunity is also true for all non-infectious diseases such as diabetes, and it applies just as strongly. The cleansing opportunity for the diabetic is given as a symbol that represents what is out of balance that needs to be rebalanced or cleansed (the non-sweetness of the life being lived that needs to be cleansed out of the life in progress). In this disease, the diabetic is given an opportunity for some deep, deep self-reflection. The diabetic can reflect on the question, "Is it sweet to exercise and keep the extra weight off to look good and be attractive to a partner?" Yes, of course it is! That is sweetness! Does the diabetic do this? Typically, no, they don't and that is at the root of their affliction.

I Do Not Fear Disease

I have reached the plateau where I am able to go through life without fearing any disease or illness. I eat a life extension diet. I exercise enough and keep fit and flexible and maintain my correct weight. I do breathwork sessions. I fast 1-day a week and periodically longer. I maintain thought patterns of wellness. I cultivate feelings of contentment, compassion and kindness. I do all of the things I know about and learn about to keep healthy in body, mind and emotions. I make and use colloidal silver if necessary. I use heat treatments in a hot soak pool or a sauna. I understand that all disease and illness offer a cleansing opportunity. And so, I do not fear disease. And I invite you to begin to move in that direction too. You can do this also! You can begin to learn to move forward in life without fearing disease. But beyond curing disease on the physical level, it is important to attain a state of always being disease free. Many things play into this including your diet, curbing your death urge, exercise, fitness, yoga, meditation, sexuality, avoiding addictions, taking better and better care of your body, providing for your life's needs, and practicing purification processes.

Life Extension Diets

SAD, is an acronym that stands for the Standard American Diet, coined by an author named Vonderplantiz, the author of two nutritional healing books that form the basis of his nutritional healing Primal Diet. The Standard American Diet (SAD), actually contributes to a wide range of health problems and shortened life spans. SAD is basically a cooked food diet. SAD is a diet with too much cooked fat. SAT is a diet with too much processed sugar. SAD is lacking in digestive enzymes. SAD contains a lot of salt. SAD often has preservatives and pesticide residues. One of the best presentations I have ever heard about the problems with SAD type diets stated that that they are nutritionally deficient, contain processed sugar, and involve cooked meats which often have antibiotic residues and contain toxins called heterocyclic amine which is found in cooked meat, and acrylamides which are found in over cooked starches. And these SAD diets often contain processed foods that contain preservatives. The presentation involved a study done on cats and dogs by a veterinarian. Her talk began with a slide show that showed published statistics which revealed that 80% of all cats die from kidney failure, and high percentage of dogs succumb to a degenerative hip disease. Of course, the food that cats and dogs are fed comes off of supermarket food shelves, and they contain preservatives and many other unnatural substances. In her presentation she told us that all of the cats and dogs under her care in her study were fed their natural raw foods that they would eat when they lived in their wild habitat. Since both cats and dogs are carnivores, the diet she fed them was raw meat. Her presentation concluded by saying that all of the animals in her study showed no disease whatsoever when fed their natural foods. So, if cats and dogs suffer degenerative diseases when they are fed processed foods, what about humans? Humans also suffer from a wide range of degenerative diseases related to SAD, such as diabetes, some forms of cancer, and it also contributes to heart disease, and to many others such as degenerative hip disease. Why is it that so many people need hip replacement? Could SAD be a factor?

There were two investigators who published books and well-known studies early in the history of processed foods and both documented the negative degenerative health effects that resulted from these SAD foods, most noticeably the rampant tooth decay that Dr. Weston Price found in his sabbatical study travels that resulted when indigenous people switched from eating their natural foods to eating processed foods. Also, the negative degenerative health effects of skeletal degeneration that Dr. Pottinger found in his five generations of cats that were fed sweet milk. What is wrong with SAD? There is deficiency of digestive enzymes and vitamins and minerals in all cooked foods. SAD contains unhealthy amounts of processed sugar found in all pastry foods and in soda pop beverages. This sugar is hard to digest and hard to utilize and eliminate and it does contribute to diabetes. SAD contains too much cooked fat which clogs the arteries with plaque and contributes to heart disease. Cooked meat contains a carcinogen (heterocyclic amine) that carries a 30% increased cancer risk. Processed, canned and packaged foods have preservatives and other questionable substances added. Finally, there is the issue of salt which contributes to high blood pressure and heart disease. And so, anyone interested in life extension should consider modifying their diet to reduce and eliminate some of these health and dietary problems.

Healthier Diets

Several diets have come on the market in recent years that offer dietary improvements. The Mediterranean Diet is often mentioned. This diet typically consists of fresh fruits, fresh vegetable salads, healthy whole grain carbohydrates in breads and cereals, healthy protein in either lean white meat, legumes, or fish, healthy fats in vegetable oil (especially olive oil), and herbs and condiments to reduce salt. Yogurt with berries, nuts and seeds, no-salt crackers with cheese and tomatoes, reduced red meat and moderate amounts of white meat, green tea, and cinnamon and unheated honey round out this diet. You will note that fast foods, processed foods, canned food, and all foods containing preservatives are omitted.

The Primal Diet

The Primal Diet is the healthiest diet that I know of. It is the basic raw food Primal Diet in the Vonderplantiz books which is very close to what our ancestors used to eat when they were hunter gathers and this diet is what humans are most compatible with and it is what our bodies are programmed for. It basically consists of raw (unpasteurized) dairy, raw (uncooked) eggs, unheated honey, fresh organic vegetable juice or hearty salads, fresh organic fruits, whole grain breads and cereals, raw (uncooked) meat, healthy oils (olive, coconut, avocado, etc.), cooked starches and legumes (beans), and unsalted, unroasted raw nuts and seeds, and also very little water. This diet is a diet for life extension and each item in it is reviewed below with comments about why it is important.

Raw Unpasteurized Dairy

Unpasteurized dairy consisting of raw milk, cream, cheese and butter is one of the main staples of this diet. It has been said that raw milk should be consumed at every meal. Raw cream is said to be the most healing food on the planet. The raw fat in raw dairy lubricates the joints and is vital for optimal cellular function. Raw butter is excellent but hard to get. Raw dairy may be hard to get for many, because in the USA it has only been legalized in 12 states as of 2022. But it is still available from 'cow share' programs in 25 other states and you can find those sources in the USA from the website www.realmilk. com. Outside the USA, there should be similar resources in your country.

Fresh Vegetable Juice or Hearty Salads

Fresh veggie juice, as everyone calls it, is at the heart of supplying abundant digestive enzymes, vitamins and minerals and it is a cornerstone health booster. It stimulates hair growth, improves hair color, stimulates fingernail and toenail growth, enriches the bloodstream with nutrients that stimulate cell function, maintains your skeletal system, promotes a feeling of wellbeing and optimal health. You should periodically check the USA government website, 'The Dirty Dozen,' to become aware of and familiar with pesticide residue levels in vegetables and fruits, but the safest way is, of course, to buy organic. Very hearty daily salads, twice daily will also suffice, but plenty of vegetables is a must.

Raw Eggs

Eggs are nature's most perfect food when eaten raw. If cooked, however, they can cause difficulties. I have heard it said that every time you eat a raw egg it slightly helps your heart, but every time you eat a cooked egg it slightly harms your heart. Raw eggs supply a raw fat that can pull out deeply buried toxins, and they are a good source of protein. An eggnog made in a blender with two or three eggs cracked right out of the shell, with a tablespoon of unheated honey and (unpasteurized) raw milk or raw cream and any fresh fruit you like is a delicious way to start eating raw eggs. However, it is much quicker to simply crack the eggs in a cup and gulp them down, and after a while you get used to it.

Fresh Fruits

Everyone knows that fresh fruits are good for you. They supply abundant nutrients and vitamins and minerals and they all taste sweet. They should be fresh, organic (if needed), and not processed in any way. It is better to eat fruits with their pulp because the pulp helps to absorb the sugar spike and keep it under control. Again, with fruits periodically check government websites. In the USA, the website, 'The Dirty Dozen,' is a good resource.

Unheated honey

Unheated honey is another powerhouse food that has the property of getting nutrients past cell membrane walls (similar to insulin) plus it has a storehouse of important digestive enzymes. All supermarket honey has been heated to prevent it from crystallizing and should be avoided. Farmer's markets are here you can find unheated honey in the USA but even there you have to be careful, because some honey sellers at farmers markets will heat their honey, and you have to ask them if it's been heated or not and get a 'no' answer. If the honey already has crystalized you know it has not been heated.

Starches and Legumes (Beans)

Organic potatoes, rice, breads, cereals and all varieties of beans and peas have always been staples but should be eaten in moderation because they can leach out vitamins and minerals. Starches and legumes supply glucose for muscle function. But many starch products, like bread, contain a wide range of preservatives and salt and sugar which should be avoided. Read the labels in breads and pick brands with very little salt or sugar or preservatives and are made with natural ingredients. There is a toxin in any starch item that has been heated and turns brown contains acrylamides. Boiled potatoes, rice and noodles contain very little acrylamides.

Vegetable Oils

Healthy vegetable oils are a good source of raw fat and raw fat is an important nutrient when it has not been heated or processed. Sources you can be sure of such as virgin olive oil are a good pick, but there are other oils, such as coconut, sunflower, grapeseed, many others. Oils should be unheated and unprocessed.

Nut and Seeds

Unsalted, unroasted sunflower seeds, pumpkin seeds, and other nuts and seeds round out the primal diet for life extension. They make a good snack food and are rich in many nutrients. But they should be unsalted and unroasted.

Concerning Meat

For most people eating meat has become a lifelong habit and is a dietary staple. But there are problems with eating meat as we will discuss below. A good approach for the life extender here would be to reduce the amount of meat you eat and switch from eating red meat to white meat and begin to reduce the white meat as the decades go by. I have read that eating meat is one of the few foods that can shorten your lifespan. This might surprise you and you might want to know why is that? Well, there are several reasons. One is that the meat from slain cows contains antibiotics to fatten them up and trace amounts of this enters the meat eater's bloodstream and this weakens the immune system. Another is that the animals that mankind eats for food are quite cogitative and know quite well what is going to happen to them when they are taken to the slaughter house and they develop a great fear and desperation over their impending death. And when humans eat this meat, that fear and desperation is still there in the aetheric field of the meat, and this fear and desperation downloads and enters the meat eater's aetheric sheath and then from there it enters the meat eater's physical body and creates a resistance and an aging effect. And the third problem with eating meat is that a carcinogen called heterocyclic amine is created whenever meat is cooked and this toxin creates, a 30% higher cancer risk for meat eaters. And last, there is the negative karmic burden that is created by eating the meat of an animal that had to be slaughtered to supply the meat. Literature exists that talks about this karmic burden and says that it can be a contributing factor in illness. A book that describes a Taoist community on top of a plateau, where some immortals lived, describes a sign at the entrance that reads, "Vegetarians Only."

Beneficial Food Combinations

I have heard that one of the causes of the weaker immune systems that humans suffer from is due to the proliferation of satellites and cell phone towers that emit 5G (5th generation) frequencies in the gigahertz range. It is said that these gigahertz frequencies create substances in the body that compromise the immune system. One nutritional combination that can combat this to some extent is to consume an avocado and an orange together at least once a week as part of your natural diet. This will help to remove some of those substances. Another food combination that is useful for ridding the body of heavy metal toxins is a combination of coconut cream and pineapple consumed before taking a 30-to-60-minute soak in hot water at 105 F.

Supplements

Supplements are not natural foods and are not well absorbed by the body. Many studies have been done on this and they always show that supplements are not well absorbed by the body. Vitamins, minerals, enzymes, and other nutritional substances that the body needs when supplied by raw vegetables and fruits are well absorbed and can be utilized efficiently by the body. The fresh, raw vegetables and fruits of your own version of the Primal Diet will supply all the vitamins, and minerals and nutrients that your body needs.

Life Extension Dietary Changes

Anyone serious about extending their life should plan on making some changes to their diet leaning towards eliminating foods that cause degeneration and foods that contain preservatives and toxins. They should begin to add foods that contain higher nutritional values. As a minimum, you should reduce cooked fats and processed sugars and add more fresh vegetables and fruits, and add more vegetable oils, such as olive oil, and add more dairy such as yogurt, and reduce processed foods, canned foods and fast-food eateries. The immortal masters I have read about have always been vegetarians. Their diet basically followed the Primal Diet. They drank raw yack milk, and consumed raw yack butter and raw yak cheese, and ate fresh vegetables, fruits, grains, legumes, cooked starches, raw eggs, and nuts and seeds.

Fasting

Anyone serious about extending their life should consider adding fasting to their life extension practices. Some people may have a hard time starting to fast 1-day a week, but recently a new fasting method called Intermittent Fasting has become quite popular and it may be an easier approach for some people to start fasting, especially for those who feel that they would not be able do a 1-day a week fast. There are several types of Intermittent Fasting.

1. The 5-2, for 2-days a week restrict calories to 500-600.

2. The 16/8 Leangrains Protocol, skip breakfast, eating restricted to 8 hours, i.e., 1-9 pm

3. Eat-Stop-Eat, fast 24 hours 1-day a week, or 2-days a week, or 3-days a week.

People who might have trouble just doing a 1-day a week fast every week may want to start with some of the easy Intermittent Fasting protocols such as the 16/8 to get over that hurdle. I have seen several people in my own circle of friends and coworkers who have achieved very impressive weight loss gains with Intermittent Fasting. However, I began with the 1-day a week fast and I had no trouble starting my own fasting practice with it, and now after 25 years, I prefer to fast 1-day a week. You just get used to it. And I have come to enjoy the break from feeding and the cleansing that it does.

Avoiding Addictions

Addictions are a major problem worldwide. Surveys suggest that at least thirty percent of all people on the planet indulge in one addiction or another. They are either overweight (sometimes very overweight), or smoke, or use alcohol, or opiates or some other drugs, recreational or pharmaceutical. Any major addiction will subtract at least ten years from your conventional life span and will, of course, negate any real chance for life extension. It is a major delusion for anyone to think they can keep on being overweight, or smoke, or drink alcohol, or use recreational drugs, and at the same time think that they can extend their life. If a person truly wants to live a longer than humans do now, but at the same time has an addiction problem, than their desire to live longer must be strong enough to overcome the addiction habit that will prevent it. Indeed, you cannot on the one hand say, "You know I like this idea of life extension – it's cool, and I'm going to go for it and extend my life," and then on the other hand, lite up a cigarette, or pour yourself an alcoholic drink, or get out a needle and shoot up some recreational drug, or eat a meal that has enough calories in it for at least three people and the cats and dogs! They simply do not go together. To become a life extender, you will need to rid yourself of addictions. Everything in the entire range of addictive substances, be it from eating too much food for the body to handle, or from smoking, or from alcohol or from recreational drugs and even some pharmaceutical drugs—are all of these are basically registered by the body as toxins. And they all undermine the body's ability to function and keep in good health. All of the underlying causes about why people use them are due to aberrant personality behavior traits that need to be healed. Deep, deep healing is needed to stop a major addiction habit.

Physical Fitness

Aerobic and Resistance Exercise

Fitness clubs have become almost the rage in recent years and those who use them are part of a large group of physically fit humans who walk the earth and they have become an almost a health-conscious sub-culture. And they show what can be done to maintain the body in a continual state of good health. There are two types of fitness exercises: aerobic and weight resistance, and both are important. Exercising in a fitness club is good because the aerobic and resistance machines are designed to minimize joint stress and also because of the convince of locker rooms and showers. Fitness experts usually say that a good fitness workout should last at least 20 minutes. Many years ago, I was told that the fitness a person gets from a good workout on one day will carry over and keep the body physically fit for two days afterwards. This means that one good workout every other day is enough. Some fitness experts recommend that an intensive hard work out should be followed the next day by an easy light work out to give the body a chance to recuperate and repair. There is a real danger in over exercising, or exercising too much. Over exercising can over stress the joints and over tax the muscles and cause injuries. Sports medicine has become common in recent years as sports injuries (and injuries caused by excessive exercising) over tax the joints, ligaments, tendons and muscles and cause tears or ruptures. It is best to exercise enough to increase fitness and benefit the body, but it is just as important to avoid injuries. A large number of sports professionals in almost any sport develop injuries over time due to the repetitive over loading of their bodies that their sport demands, and this even applies to some of the performing arts such as ballet. When you exercise, fitness clubs are desirable, but if a fitness club is not available (such as during COVID-19) you can still exercise outdoors and jog, or speed walk, or go up and down stairs or trails or hills, or do aerobic movements and calisthenics in place, all of which will keep you physically fit and healthy.

Yoga Postures and Movements

It has been said that most people do not maintain enough flexibility and suppleness in their bodies and that this contributes to aging. Indeed, there are many older yoga fitness practitioners who look much younger than their years. The body needs to kept flexible and supple. There is nothing like the relief from aches and pains that you get after a good yoga workout. Many common aches and pains that people complain about can be eliminated or substantially reduced through yoga posture movements. You can do yoga movements outdoors such as the salutation-to-the-sun and keep yourself flexible. I do all three: aerobic, resistance, and yoga movements. When I lapse on one, I notice it. When these three types of exercises and movements are done on a relatively regular basis, your resulting health becomes quite good. And it keeps your immune system strong enough to ward off most diseases. All three of these types of exercises and movements will help you stay physically fit and extend your life.

Take Better and Better Care of Your Physical Body

This is an important aspect of your journey into a very long life that is often overlooked. You will need to take better and better care of your physical body and treat it as if it is the most precious thing that you own because it is—it is what allows you to be here. It is very important to give your body the very best care you can. And when you give your body the very best care, it can last and last and last. Always give your body the best foods you can afford. Vegetables and fruits should always be organic (if needed, check the 'Dirty Dozen' website) and fresh. There is no substitute for dental care, and your teeth need to be cleaned and maintained on a regular basis. New products keep coming on the market such as the water pic for cleaning teeth and gums and it is wise learn about them and use them. Your body needs to be cleansed regularly. It needs regular showers. Your body is designed to be used. Daily activity is needed. You will need to keep your body healthy. Your body needs to be kept free of disease. Any disease you get needs to be healed. You will need to provide for your life necessities: a place to live, a car, food, clothes, etc. You will need to have an income to support all of this. I'm sure it is a sad truism that homeless people most likely will not be extending their life.

Totally missing from our civilization is this – 'the natural human life span is 140-150 years.'

Indeed, and in a few places in the world there are humans who do reach it.

CHAPTER 3
Life Extension Affirmations

Oh, Life extension – it's in the power of your mind – it's key
To a much longer life span – this is the future human legacy.
But enmeshed as we are in the mass consensus belief
In aging and death – we live and age and die in grief
With lives of struggle, stress and trouble without relief.
But if you can attain higher consciousness enough to know
That your life can flow on with ease and joy then you can go
For life extension, and you can go for anyway it even though
The masses lag behind until they too evolve enough to find
That they have the same ability as everyone to be aligned
To the higher spectrum thoughts and emotions of the kind
That adores creation with all of its life abounding all around –
And abhors war, wanting world brotherhood to be found –
And uses compassionate action in ways that do astound!
If you can create thoughts and beliefs that allow you to arrive
At life extension, and if that way of life becomes what you create
Through your affirmations and life pattern changes then I'll state
That this indeed sets the stage to let your lifespan really soar
Well past 150 years and even go beyond for many years more!

Your Natural Potential Life Span is 140 to 150 Years

From many different voices, some speaking to audiences, others writing articles and books, and a few speaking to me in dreams, I heard it said over and over again—that in this New Age of Aquarius, beginning Dec 21, 2012, it will become possible to live twice as long as before. This means that if you begin to allow that idea to come into your consciousness and belief system, you can expect to live 140 to 150 years! I found this highly exciting. As soon as I heard about it, I wanted to learn how do it. And so, I began to gather more and more information about this idea of life extension. This may seem like a huge stretch because you have never heard of anyone who has lived anywhere near that long. And yet, Wikipedia has articles that list 100 of the world's oldest men and women and each and every one of them was over 110! And this list even included humans who were over 114! There are probably at least 500 men and women now living on the earth who are over 110. And so, it is possible to live to a ripe old age and none of the people in those lists knew anything about the practices and procedures of longevity and life extension that you will read about and learn in this book.

And starting around 2016 this idea of life extension has gained great momentum worldwide as organizations such as the RAAD Fest have sprung up. RAAD stands for Revolution Against Aging and Death and it presents major medical science antiaging breakthroughs and the latest age reversal technologies from many areas of science. And the RAAD Fest organization and others like it have held major events in many metropolitan areas around the world and these are slowly beginning to have an effect on the mass conscious reality belief system about how long a human can live.

What if today's supercentenarians had used and applied the practices of the life extender that you will read about here? Could not they have reached the 140 to 150 years of the natural lifespan of a human being? They probably could have! And they might have been able to go past that 140 to 150 benchmark as well. And what about the masters of physical immortality? Although very few have ever heard of them or believe that they exist, they are there, and indeed the practices of the masters when utilized opens up a real potential for physical immortality – and now I'm talking about living over 300 years and even past 500 years! And the techniques of the Taoist Immortals (some, of whom lived through many Chinese dynasties) will be revealed in the last chapter of this book. Yes, indeed, the secrets of the immortals will be revealed!

At the most fundamental level, I learned that longevity has to do with the power of your mind. I learned that if you do not expect to age you will not age like everyone else does. You won't age as fast as the masses trapped in the mass consensus reality belief system about aging. But there are many, many other things that play into longevity and life extension. You will also need to learn how to go forward in life without fearing that you could get some horrible disease. In addition, you will need to learn the importance feeling the positive emotions of compassion and benevolence and love. You will need to shut off negative media thought programming and orient your thought patterns into the creative expectations of the life extender. You will need to heal your death urge. You should practice the longevity breathing techniques. You should consider incorporating fasting. And sexuality has a role to play in longevity and life extension.

Occasionally I like to ask someone how long they think they are going to live. Usually they will say something like, "Oh, my mother died at 90, and I think that that's about how long I'll live." And they also think that when you're that old you will be a decrepit, weak and wobbly, crinkled and crumpled, frail and fragile old wreck, and what fun can life possibly be after you get to be that old? Well, they are assuming that they will age just like the older people all around them have always done. But it's possible to change all that and we will begin to reveal how you can do that. We should state that there are many older people who do look good, who are fit and attractive, and who have kept their vitality, and who do look in their later years like mature vital people. And for most of you, your older years can be your best. I like to ask the same person later on, "Well, what if it were possible for you to get rejuvenated so that you would look and feel like you were forty or fifty again?" When they hear that they usually say, "All right, sign me up! Where do I go? I'll be the first in line to get rejuvenated!"

I learned that at the most foundational level, life extension will have to do with the power of your mind. I learned that if you do not expect to age you will not age as fast as everyone else does. If you are able to cultivate this belief system, this expectation, that you are not going to age as fast as the masses, that you are going to age much more slowly, then you won't age as fast as the masses do. You won't age as fast as they do because they are entrained in the mass consensus reality belief system about aging, but you will need to free yourself from all of that. I learned that we all have an aging program set up in our minds linked to our culture that creates an expectation to age in a certain fashion the way everyone else does. This aging program creates what the masters call premature aging. I also learned that your preponderant thought patterns are fundamentally a product of your belief system, and they follow what you expect will happen, and what you think you deserve, and what you think is possible. In order to support life extension, your beliefs about how long a human can live will need to change and expand. What you expect to happen is what tends to happen. Your belief system is also based upon what you think is possible or not possible. If you think life extension, or living to 140–150 is impossible, then it is.

Your thoughts follow your beliefs and so you will need to expand your beliefs about what you think is possible or not possible. In addition, your thoughts also are coupled with what you think you deserve. It is important to begin to formulate the idea that you certainly do deserve to live that long. And fundamentally, to really create life extension, (to actualize it, or actually do it) you will need to create an expectancy of it. This involves expecting that you are going to extend your life span with a certain cockiness. You eventually will come to the point where you just know it is going to happen. Then it becomes a knowingness or knowledge. You just know you are going to do it because you have learned how to do it and that is all there is to it. You create a foundational, fundamental expectation that you know you are going to do it. And then you will need to plan on it. And as time goes by, you will just need to allow it to happen. You simply let it happen because it will.

Of course, this goes against current beliefs systems about how long a human can live, and therefore you will need to counter the life expectancy beliefs of your culture. It is suggested that you work with the many, many affirmations, meditations, visualizations, and practices of the life extender that you will read about in this book. Every time you work with and master a life extension affirmation, or a life extension breathing pattern, or a life extension fasting routine, or a life extension meditation or visualization exercise, it adds to your belief system or your tool box of life extension beliefs, and this greatly helps you counter the beliefs of your culture. We will repeat this, it is that important. Every time you master a new affirmation or technique or life extension life style change, it adds another tool to your master tool box of life extension beliefs. Another very strong technique you can use to counter the status que life expectancy is to use fanaticism. Quietly become a fanatic about it. But don't shout it out to others, because they will try to give you their beliefs of the current longevity status quo. But internally and quietly create and maintain a determined, dominant, unshakeable, fanatical mindset that you are a life extender period, and you are going to do it, and that is all there is to it, and nothing is going to change that! And then make it a dominant intention of yours. You should cultivate the expectation that you are going to extend your life and there is nothing in the world that is going to stop you from doing it, period!

It is important to know that "The Universal Law of Thought," is one of the twelve universal laws, and is at the heart of what you create. The Universal Law of Thought says, "Thought is the creative force of the universe." Mankind basically uses thought in a negative way and this is apparent in the worldwide health problems of the human race. Those of higher consciousness talk about the power of thought in a very deep and systematic way. They speak about the importance of creating thought patterns of on-going continual health. And they talk about the problems that negative thoughts create. They talk about thought-forms that are created whenever someone creates an image (or imagines or visualizes an idea). They say that the thought-form is a created entity in and of itself and it attaches to the one who created it, and it wants and tries to impulse its creator to carry out the intent of whatever the thought was about.

Those of higher consciousness also talk about the importance of maintaining positive emotions. And they speak about the importance of creating emotional patterns of harmony and contentment. And they talk about the wide spectrum of health problems that negative emotions create. Learning how to maintain positive emotions is also a very important part of life extension.

Your culture and the internet and the media enmesh people in what might be called the mass consensus reality belief systems about basically everything in life and it tends to be on the negative side. There are some news stories now about greater longevity, but by and large it is a good idea to become as media free as you can. When you do this, it is much easier on your belief system to create and nurture your own beliefs about becoming a life extender. There are groups involved in life extension and it would be very a good idea to join them.

There are many practices and process for life extension in this book that will help you to establish thought patterns of extending your life. The more you work with all of the affirmations, meditations, visualization exercises, and the other processes and practices in this book (and in others) to extend your life, the easier it will be for you to create the belief system that you can do it and are going to do it and go for it. This is because they will all feed into your belief system and then you will begin to believe that it makes more and more sense that you can do this.

It is appropriate here to look at what the average potential life span of a human is. Most people would say (because of their mass consensus reality belief system programming) that a human can live around 90 to 100 years. But I was given a very powerful dream a few years ago that completely contradicts this. For several weeks I had been wanting an answer to the question, "How long is the natural potential life span of a human?" And then I was given a dream in which a voice (a kind but firm voice) spoke very plainly and said,

"At this point in time, a human can live in good health and acuity for 140 to 150 years. It is possible to extend further [using life extension techniques] to 200 to 250 years, but to go much beyond that would require a change to your whole civilization allowing for much more benevolent systems to evolve."

So, I believe that your natural potential life span is 140 to 150 years. And I believe that life extension is going beyond that – going for 200 to 250 years.

So Why Don't Humans Live 140 to 150 Years?

Many will find it hard to believe that their natural potential lifespan is 140 to 150 years because they will say that no one lives that long. Even those who maintain a high fitness level or practice very healthy life styles don't make it much over 100, if they live that long. So, this begs the question that if your potential life span is 140 to 150, what is it that causes humans fall 40 to 50 years short of that?

I was given another dream some years later after I had been intently thinking about this question for several days, "Why don't humans live long enough to reach their natural potential lifespan?" Again, in the dream, I heard a voice speak, and I was shown visions.

"Humans on earth have some damage to their major organs: liver, kidneys, lungs, pancreas, etc. And if humans were able to love each other more, especially with family members, then their own health problems would not as severe [and they could live longer]. Nutritional healing diets are helpful, and supportive and nurturing groups are healing."

I think this is one of the reasons why people don't make it anywhere near their potential life span. But again, I think that the most important reason is the mass consensus reality belief system that says that people can only live 90 to 100 years. Another major factor is what the immortals called the 'death urge.' Elderly people, when they find themselves advanced in age and discover that old people are left out of mainstream society simply decide that they don't want to continue on. There are also many other factors that contribute to aging and death. Some of these are: succumbing to a major disease, aging caused by addictions, aging caused by the body clock and the death hormone release, and aging caused by soul fragmentation. And as the dream said, damage to the major organs takes a toll on human longevity.

The dream also pointed out that the ability to love each other more then we as a culture are able to do now is the way to heal this. Therefore healing – deep healing, is the next major step to attaining life extension. And after that, it is important to raise to higher levels of consciousness. In addition, much has recently been revealed to humanity in new information and techniques and spiritual technologies on how to live longer and extend your life. You will read about all about all of this in later chapters.

The Human Body Is Actually Designed to Live Over 200 Years

You will start to hear this from many different sources that humans are designed to live over 200 years and even much longer than that and then humans will finally start to believe it, and then accept it, and then actually begin to live it. It is very important to know that short life spans are from false programming and low fear consciousness, and this is all part of the old paradigm, part of the old dark energy prior to 2012, part of the Age of Pisces. But all of this is changing as we are slowly moving into the new age of Aquarius, and as we incorporate the new energy of compassion, benevolence and integration, and slowly people will want to start living longer and longer, and as they learn how to do it, they will learn that it will mostly have to do developing the expectancy that living at least 200 years is the new norm.

In December of 2020, I was given another very powerful dream after I had been intently thinking for several days about the rejuvenating aspects of a series of 1-hour exposures to trace levels of the slightly radioactive gas, radon, and in the dream a voice said,

"By adding [periodic] radon healing radiation treatments, I could go for 230 years [instead of only 200]."

In other words, the dream told me that I could add another 30 years by incorporating periodic radon gas radiation healing treatments. What this says is that these life extension practices, process, treatments and therapies are additive. This means that when you add and master another one, more years of an extended life span can become possible for you.

The Affirmations

My first experience with the practices of physical immortality or life extension were with the affirmations. The traditional training practices of physical immortality started with and were centered around the affirmations. The physical immortality training workshops that I took were always done in a group setting and this adds more power. The affirmations were always said out loud, and with a real zeal. The twenty to forty of us in the group would sit in chairs arranged around in a large circle. Each person would read out loud one of the affirmations and add his or her name in the gap after the initial 'I'. The next person would read the next affirmation and so on until all of the affirmations were read out loud around the circle. At the end of each affirmation the Sanskrit word 'Ja' (pronounced like the letter 'J') was shouted in exhilaration to add excitement, enthusiasm and exuberance to the affirmation.

Traditional affirmations for physical immortality

1. I,   , know that the divine alchemist within is transforming the appearance of my body to express its eternal longevity and its eternal youthfulness. Ja!

2. I,   , know that my physical body is my natural universe over which I alone rule. It is my material sheath which I am continually remanifesting through the powers of the divine nature of my mind. My physical body is my servant and although perishable, I am continually renewing it. Ja!

3. I,   , am rapidly progressing in mastering the higher dimensional physics, and I know that I can recreate my body's form into the ageless expression of a mature, vital, immortal human. Ja!

New Life Extension Affirmations

However, in our day much has changed. I have created a whole new set of affirmations that incorporate the new information. Modern practices for cultivating a life extension belief system use a series of affirmations to program the subconscious mind which will in turn influence the conscious mind to create a new belief system for life extension. Life extension is possible and we just need to work on creating it. Life extension is, indeed, a real potential.

For the new life extension affirmations, I feel that the practice of adding the exclamatory 'Ja!' or any other such exclamation such as 'yes!' or 'right on!' or, 'you got that right!' is optional. I have included them in some of the affirmations, but omitted them from most of the others in the list below. But if you want to use them you can be creative and add any exclamatory phrase you choose, such as: "Yes, yes that is right!" Or you can use modern slang, if you like, such as: "Right on!", or "You bet!"

You will need to work with these affirmations. If you can do them in a group setting it will add more energy and influence to your affirmation sessions, but if you can't (and most of the time you won't be able to), you will still need to say them on your own. You will get great benefit from them on your own and they will immensely help lead you to your own longevity and life extension belief system. Say each affirmation out loud but in a low voice and let the meaning and the intent of each affirmation resonate deeply within you. When you do this, you will receive benefit from each one of them. You should make it a point to say each of them.

And then after you've gone through the whole list, you should pick one or two that you really resonate to and say it every day. Yes, every single day! One of them should be an affirmation for extending your life. It is best to say your affirmations the first thing every morning as soon as you get out of bed and your feet hit the floor. But, if you forget to say them in the morning, then say them later as soon as you remember that you forgot to say them. And as time goes on and you become adept at your own work in extending your life, you will probably want to create some new life extension affirmations that you know will be specifically designed and oriented just for you and your own life circumstances.

Why Are Life Extension Affirmations So Important?

At this slice in time (10 years past 2012) life extension affirmations are at the heart of conditioning your belief system because life extension is not supported by the mass conscious reality belief system at this time, and those of us who are going to extend our lives will need to create our own belief system that does support it. And life extension affirmations are at the heart of this. In ten generations beyond 2012 (that is 200 beyond 2012), predictions are that the population at large will start to see large numbers of people living 150 years and beyond, and by then many will just come to expect it, and then they will begin to live it because it will have become the new norm.

There was an article about the life span expectancy of children who lived in a mountainous district of Peru where many of the people were very long-lived. These children were asked how long they thought they would live, and all of them said, "well, at least 110, maybe 120...," because living that long was the experience and expectancy of the majority of the people. And since the children identified with their villagers who were living 'at least 110,' they began to create an expectancy of at least matching it in their own belief systems. And that really is the key to life extension.

In our current time now (a decade after 2012), life extension affirmations along with a powerful determination to extend your life are needed to overcome the bias of our civilization at large. It is well to study fanatism in regard to this. Fanatics make their reality real due to their fanatical, zealous approach to it. In like manner we too can benefit from being just a little bit fanatical about our will to become a life extender. In being a fanatic about life extension, I mean being a fanatic internally. I do not recommend being a fanatic about it in public or at your workplace for obvious reasons. Also note that in our first basic affirmation below, '...I am a life extender...,' note that the 'I am a life extender' has special meaning for a life extender because it says that if you currently have some physical health problems that you will find a way to cure them or overcome them.

You need to speak these affirmations out loud in a low voice. Find a place and time where you won't be disturbed to do this. The Universal Law of Speech says, "Speech will be used to influence." Allow your speech when you say an affirmation to influence your subconscious mind where it will influence your conscious mind and reality. When you speak an affirmation let the words really sink in. When you say your affirmation that you are going to extend your life, let that sink in and begin to accept that you are really are going to extend your life. When you say your affirmation that you are going to live 140–150 years, begin to accept that this as a real potential for you, and begin to plan on it. Let the meaning of words become real. Begin to own the affirmations you speak. And as time goes on, pick the affirmations to speak that state your own truth. Remember, an affirmation is something that you affirm that you are going to do. It is what you plan on doing. And so, begin to accept that and allow it. And the more you say your affirmations, the more they cognate as your real future potential. Go deeper and deeper with your affirmations as time goes on and begin to plan your life around your affirmations.

Also, you should say more than just one affirmation and you should vary your affirmations. As one affirmation in our list below becomes a little old, change it for another one in the list. But one of your daily affirmations every day should focus on extending your life.

Affirmations for Beginning Life Extension

1. I am a life extender. I am going to extend my life and that is all there is to it!

2. I have heard that the natural potential lifespan of all humans is 140 to 150 years at the current level of consciousness, and I'm going to go for it. Yes, I am!

3. I, as a life extender, am going to go for my natural potential life span of 140 to 150 years! And I know that if my conviction is strong enough about it, then it does not matter if everyone else thinks you can't live that long. My conviction is strong enough to do it, and I'm going to do it, and that is all there is to it!

4. I fully understand and cognate what it means when I affirm that I am going to go for a life span of 140 to 150 years. It means that I am going to plan on doing it. It means that I am going to plan on adding the many, many years that I will need to reach my life span goal to be here and see the year 2060 or 2080 or 2100. I fully understand that this is what it means when I say my affirmation to go for 140 to 150 years.

5. I know that life extension affirmations are very important to change my beliefs about how long a person can live, and to repattern my belief system so that my new beliefs are those of a life extender. And, I intend to say my daily affirmation to extend my life the very first thing every morning as soon as I get out of bed and my feet hit the floor! I intend to do this every day without fail. And if I miss a morning, I will say it later in the day. Oh yes, Indeed I will!

6. I am going to say good riddance to my death urges, and say, "I welcome my on-going life urges, and all of the good things in life that I intend to have come my way to enjoy and look forward to every day in my very long life."

7. I, as a life extender, intend to conquer my death urge. Every day my life becomes more interesting, more creative, and more exciting, so much so that I just want to stay here and live a lot longer. Yes!

8. I practice maintaining my body in good health and fitness and flexibility through physical exercise and yoga workouts as I feel I need to. Yes, I do!

9. I will deal with and correct all of my health issues!

10. I will move to better and better nutritional diet that supports life extension.

11. I am learning the cure and the prevention of all disease. Right on!

12. I intend to avoid all addictions including overeating, smoking, drinking alcohol, and recreational and some pharmaceutical drugs. You bet!

13. I, as a life extender, intend to deal with and overcome any addiction tendencies or traits I may have, including overeating. Yes, I will!

14. I understand and work with the power of the breath. I am beginning to start my breath work practices. I am also beginning to breathe deeper throughout my daily activities. Yes, Indeed I am!

15. I understand the benefits of Intermittent Fasting and the 1-day a week fast. I am beginning to start my fasting practices now. Yes, I am!

16. I understand and work with the power of the affirmations, and visualization-meditations for life extension, and I intend to do them and incorporate them. Indeed!

17. I am learning to take better and better care of my precious physical body in all ways: physically, emotionally, mentally and financially, and to treat my body as if it is the most precious thing I own, because it is, it is what allows me to be here. Exactly!

18. I know that at the most fundamental level that all I have to do to live longer is to make an intention to extend my life – but I know that this means that I will consciously incorporate everything that allows it to happen and get rid of everything else that will stop it from happening. I absolutely will!

19. I, as a life extender, know that all illness and degeneration can be healed and on a daily basis I work with what my body needs most to keep it balanced and healed.

20. I, as a life extender, intend to wean myself away from early planned death that is continually bombarded at us from Medicare, life insurance, funeral homes and the like. I refuse to plan for my death by not getting involved with any of this. I plan on extending my life and that is all there is to it!

21. I, as a life extender, will do my daily life extension affirmations. And I will exercise if I need it. And I will adopt a life extension diet of my own choosing. And I will create on-going life extension thoughts and emotional patterns. Yes, I know that all of this is very important for extending my life.

22. I, as a life extender, know that antiaging and age reversal technologies are ballooning right now and I intend to take advantage of some of them that I feel may help me extend my life when they become available.

23. I know that part of life extension is to have a purpose in life and I continually work on creating a meaningful purpose for my life. I know that there are plenty of things out there that need to change to make our word a better place and I will choose those that are the most meaningful and important for me to get involved in and help make these needed changes happen. Indeed!

24. I practice ongoing dietary purification, ridding toxins, and adding food and drink of high nutritional value that support life extension. Oh, yes!

What Are Most Important Things You Need to Do to Reach 140 to 150 Years?

The items below are what I think are the most important things you should do to reach for the goal of extending your life, or of going for a 140-to-150-year life span.

1. **Say Your Daily Affirmations that State that You Are Going to Extend Your Life**

Daily every morning as soon as you get out of bed and your feet hit the floor you should say one or more daily affirmations for life extension. And at night when you are getting ready for bed say in a low loving voice that you want the extra oxygen and prana from your breathwork to trigger the regeneration of new cells. One of the affirmations I often use is, "I am going to extend my life and that is all there is to it!" But what does that mean? It means that you are going to do all of the things that you know will help you live longer in all areas and aspects of your life. If it appears you need to get more exercise, then you will decide that you need to do it and then you will do it. It means that if you know you need to move to a better diet more suited to greater longevity then you will do that. It means that if you know you should take some action to improve your health you will do it.

I would suggest adding an additional affirmation that states a specific longevity goal such as, "My dominant intention is to reach my potential life span of 140 to 150 years, and I'm going to go for it!" I would reflect to you here that you should select an age goal that you think you could actually reach. If you come up with something like 300 years, and you know your health isn't up to it, then your belief system won't support it. But if you think you could make it to 110, then choose that as your goal, and then your belief system will believe that your goal is possible and then it will reflect something back to you like this to all of your body cells and systems, "Ok, our owner wants us live at least 110 years, so let's get all of our body parts and pieces working together in perfect harmony and balance to let that happen." As time goes on, you should say several affirmations a day, perhaps throughout the day, and pick new ones from the list that you don't usually say. Eventually you may want to create a new affirmation that is exactly prevalent and pertinent for you. You should eventually strive to create the unshakeable life extension mindset a – LIFE EXTENSION MINDSET - through this constant reminder that life extension is what you are going to go for and there is nothing in this world that is going to stop you from doing it. That in my opinion is the most important thing you need to do.

2. Deal With Whatever Addictions You May Have

Statistics on addictions reveal that 30% of the world's population has one addiction or another and they will all subtract years from your life span. And the top addiction on my list is overeating. Do not kid yourself, overeating is an addiction and it is a problem worldwide. If this is a problem of yours it is very important for you to overcome it if you want to extend your life. And all of the other addictions need to be avoided as well. I have watched many people go into an early decline and death at an early age because of their addictions.

3. Conquer Your Death Urge

Indeed, many older people feel that the world is oriented to the young (and there is a lot of truth in this) and they feel left out, and this takes a big toll on their desire to want continue their lives. It is very important to create a life that you want to continue. Add the missing recreation and entertainment that you enjoy. If a partnership is missing or has been lost it is important to find new relationships to stimulate and sustain you. Let your creativity burst forth. Create the things you love. Daily, make life enjoyable enough so that you want to continue on. Become one who really enjoys life.

4. Add Breathwork and Fasting

Although it is not absolutely necessary, breathwork can add a great deal of oxygen and life force energy into your body for enhanced healing, regeneration and youthing. The life extension aspirant should consider adding some breathwork to their life extension activities. The same is true for fasting. Intermittent Fasting is popular now and it works for many people it may be a way that works for you to add fasting to your life extension practices. Many have found that Intermittent Fasting helps them keep their weight under control. But for those who can do the 1-day a week fast every week and occasional add longer fasts, that would be a better choice to begin fasting.

5. Add More Compassion, Love, Light and Joy

Become kinder every day. Daily go out of your way to make others smile and feel happier and enjoy chatting with you. Avoid like the plague getting into or drawn into condemning and derogative conversations with others. Weekly work with compassion and gratitude and the healers. Daily begin to feel and work with the increasing light that is coming to planet and choosing to feel joy and happiness more and more often. Notice how all of this helps you enjoy your day and your life more. And note that these tools for extending your life all work together.

6. Learn to Live Without Fearing Disease

I have helped two people heal themselves from cancer and I know that all afflictions and illnesses can be healed. I periodically take note of my own physical condition and find the areas that I need to work on and heal, and I work on them. I use the natural healing facilities that I know of such as the hot spring resorts and the radon health mines. For bacterial and viral infections, I use natural remedies such as colloidal silver, herbal remedies and heat. Other important areas to work on that are not so obvious are the many emotional wounds that you have suffered, and the emotional tendencies you may have that irritate others, and the negative mental thought patterns that greatly affect and impact your health and longevity. It is important to acknowledge and own them and then work on healing them like the Master from Galilee taught so well several thousand years ago. And it is important also to know that some afflictions, such as cancer have to do with not having learned a soul life lesson, such as learning to stop verbally whiplashing a fellow soul brother or sister that appears in some cases of lung and throat cancer. And other afflictions such as dementia may have to do with not having learned the soul lesson of being able to stop over mentalizing, and to allow the emotional and physical sides of the three-sided triangle of beingness to be expressed instead of mentally suppressing them as is seen in some cases of dementia. I do not fear disease. It is important for a life extender to begin to also not fear disease.

7. Keep Fit

Some form of daily exercise is needed. Keeping active is important. Fitness clubs are good. The body needs to be used and maintained. Good exercise workouts on a regular basis can actually keep you free of many diseases. People have been cured from heart disease and diabetes through regular resistance and aerobic exercises. Yoga movements and stretching keep the body flexible and maintained and have helped heal many common chronic aches and pains throughout the body. All of these can help you live longer. But be careful to avoid injury due to over exercise.

8. Move to a Better Diet

You should begin shift away from the Standard American Diet (SAD) into a diet more suited to longevity and life extension as the years go by. The diets mentioned here will help to supply the nutrients and energy needed for ongoing regeneration and can supply the optimal nutritional needs that your body has. Also, add fasting, perhaps Intermittent Fasting to for weight control.

9. Put an Important Purpose in your Life

It is important to devote your life to the things that are so important for us all as one human family on the earth. We need to have our world transformed into a place of peace and harmony and benevolence. So there are many things that need to be changed and some of them are things that you can get involved in and help to make happen. The list is a long one, such as helping to put an end to homelessness, helping to stop the human created 6th mass extension, helping to put an end to racial prejudice, etc. etc., etc. and all of you can pick the things most important to you and help to make them happen. And this will help you too – it will give you a purpose for continuing your life journey into life extension.

10. Commit to Reaching an Extended Life Span or Your Natural Potential of 140-150 Years

Every day feel it happening. Make little changes, small adjustments in your life on a regular basis that will allow you to move closer and closer to a person who is going to do it. You should periodically go through all of the affirmations. You should add and create new affirmations for yourself as you grow into becoming a life extender. If you need a better diet, you should go for it. If you need more exercise, you should do it. If you need more social life, you should allow yourself to be available for it. If you need a partner, do what it takes to attract a partner. If you need more income, create the abundance you need. But every day you should begin to create the thought patterns that you are becoming a life extender, and as we say, "that is all there is to it!"

Recap on the Most Important Things to do to Extend Your Life

To reach your potential life span of 140 to 150 years should not be that hard really. For those who are in their 40s or 50s, it will mean adding 100 more years to their life. Basically, this will involve avoiding the premature aging program, and it will require you to keep yourself free of disease. This basically means that you plan on living without the need for disease. All you really need to do is simply live like you are going to live to at least 140 or 150 years of age. And it means you intend to do it! What you intend to do, you do! It means you put in place all of the things you know about or learn about that will help you to live longer. It means you will avoid all of the things you know will harm you or hobble your quest for life extension. It means you plan on doing it. It means you will work on avoiding the aging belief of the masses. It means you will keep yourself fit and flexible and healthy. It means you will avoid retiring into a life of doing nothing but play because you know that that will tend to signal your end. You will create a purpose or a goal for all of your years including what is considered today as your retirement years. It means you welcome change. It means you plan on supporting yourself financially for at least 140 to 150 years.

Is It Necessary to Do the Breathwork and Fasting to Extend Your Life?

The short answer is 'no' they are not absolutely necessary to extend your life. But the longer answer is that doing them, even occasionally, will help you greatly to change your belief system and that is one of the real keys. This is needed because you are going against the mass conscientious reality belief about human life expectancy. But it also needs to be strongly emphasized that the benefits you can receive from the breathwork and the fasting are also very real and are also a major part of helping you to extend your life because they are directly involved in helping you stay healthy and living longer and adding more energy, and purifying your body. There are many other very important factors for creating life extension that you will read about in later chapters: low DNA efficiency, the body clock and death hormone release, soul fragmentation, past life bias, and more. And so, when you work with the visualization-meditations to heal them, this will also influence your belief system and this will give you a greater impetus for actually extending your life. The visualization-meditations can heal and raise your consciousness level and bring more life force energy in and all of this will help you extend your life. And it is the same for breathwork and fasting. So, all of the practices and exercises and meditations are additive and work together and all of them will influence your belief system and heal your body and bring in more energy and get rid of toxins and as such, all of them can help take you further into extending your life. But the short answer is 'no, breathwork and fasting' are not absolutely necessary to extend your life, but doing them is very helpful for extending your life, and so the long answer is 'yes, they are helpful and they can help you to go further with a greater extension of your life if you will do them and all of the other life extension practices in this book.'

The ancient masters of immortality did not fear disease.

Part 2

Intermediate Practices of Life Extension

Your Body Can Actually Live Over 300 Years

I've heard many say your basic human body design is for you to live far longer than your current potential natural lifespan of 140-150 years, and it is important to note that they also say that your body is actually designed to give you a life span of over 300 years. Yes, over 300 years and some of the masters of physical immortality have demonstrated it. Your body is capable of many things (telepathy is another) that your science doesn't recognize as possible.

CHAPTER 4
Heal, Heal, Heal

Oh, what it is that undermines human health the most?
It is disease, and if you please, ponder on the remedy
And you will see the remedy is free – completely free,
This remedy is love from above or from you the host.
Love is the healer – even if an illness is diagnosed
Love is being wanted, taken care of, being adored
Love is wanting happiness for all – that is your reward!

Why don't people live long enough to reach their natural lifespan of 140 to 150 years? There are many reasons for this, but one of them, a major one, is that they succumb to one disease or another. When the body is kept in the balanced state – emotionally, mentally, physically, and even in the traits of the soul – then there is no disease, and there is no need for disease. This implies that disease is something that is out of balance. And so, the next step is to look at how any disease can be restored back into balance.

One of the most profound statements I have ever heard about our human civilization was that the number one most important thing that all men and women need is deep healing. It is hard to understate this. It is also hard to fully appreciate what this really means since we are in a world where struggle, lack, separation and the many, many gaps is the standard fare and experience. There are gaps between the will of the people and the intention of the politicians, gaps between the haves and the have nots (from those supported by the economic engines and those who are not). There are gaps in housing and food availability, the application of justice and policing, health care and coverage. There are many others gaps that exist in politics, religions, education, etc. These gaps all create conflict and result in a sort of resentment and distrust, and believe it or not, this causes some of the underlying health issues that people suffer from that are hard to define, but exist nonetheless.

It is axiomatic that deep healing is the most needed thing on the planet. Indeed, if the majority of the human race were steeped in this, I doubt that the atrocities that you read about in the news would happen. Love and compassion are said to be the greatest healers of all. Feeling love for others and sending love out to others is at the heart of helping to heal them and yourself. Being able to feel love for yourself and to send love to yourself is the basis of healing yourself on all levels. Fear and stress and resentment are at the opposite poles of the healing spectrum. They are causes of disease.

I have heard it said that Master Jesus required those who he healed to answer two questions before he would heal them. The first was, "Do you want to be healed?" While this might sound obvious, many people want their health problems because they know that it brings them attention that they would not get otherwise, and the attention was what they really wanted. So, in order for Jesus to heal them permanently they would have to fully accept that being healed was what they really wanted. The second question was, "Will you give your life over to God?" He asked them that because he knew that they created their disease in the first place, and they would likely recreate it unless they were willing to give their life over to a higher power.

Now let us look at deep healing. Deep healing involves being able to rise above the gaps, to accept things the way they are, and to work with the traditional practices – the six perfections, and with the more modern processes that I have termed the nine deep healers. Deep healing also is connected to developing a knowledge of the Twelve Universal Laws. The Infinite Creator gave its creation twelve creative principles which are usually called the Twelve Universal Laws and learning about them and working with them is part of healing and higher consciousness and even life extension.

The Six Perfections

The masters in the tradition of the Buddhists Monasteries of the far east were said to teach their disciples a number of practices for developing higher consciousness. These practices were called the Six Perfections. They are:

1. Generosity
2. Patience
3. Tolerance
4. Concentration
5. Joyful effort
6. Wisdom

In this training, the students were given one of the six perfections to study and work on each week and at the end of the six weeks they would know and would have worked with all six of them. For the 'generosity' week, the students would focus on everything that happened to them that invoked a feeling of being generous, especially for the gift of life. They were coached to say things like, "Thank you," after receiving something – a gift, a kind word, a helpful suggestion, and the like. They were coached to notice everything that invoked a feeling of generosity in them and then they were asked to write down these occurrences so that they would not forget them. At the end of the week there would be an around the room sharing and each in turn would speak about and relate their experiences of feeling generous.

It would be good to emulate this because these steps are the beginning steps to reaching higher consciousness and this will help you to attain life extension. For one week pick one of them to work with it and write down where it is hard for you and where it is easy. It would be best to do this with a group, but you can do it on your own. This list is good because it gets at things that many people have difficulty with and need to work on, such as patience, tolerance, and concentration. For one week work on each of these in turn.

Generosity

Work on being generous, and that can include giving someone a smile, a helpful suggestion, or giving them some of your time. It does not have to be elaborate or expensive.

Patience

Work on patience, and notice when you are impatient and then command yourself to become patient in all situations where you feel entrapped in a world rushing by to get somewhere in a hurry.

Tolerance

Work on becoming more tolerant and pay close attention to the people or situations that you find yourself intolerant of and try to get at root cause and then work on letting it go, just letting it go.

Concentration

Work on developing greater concentration. Begin to look at the times that you are scattered and cannot focus. Concentrate and focus on objects and symbols and try to hold those images for several minutes. Concentrating on a candle flame is traditional. After several minutes students were asked to close their eyes and visualize the candle after image in their mental screen for as long as they could.

Joyful effort

Work at being joyful in the tasks that you do during the week. Work on feeling that the task you are doing is needed and is helping someone or something or the earth and find joy in doing the task.

Wisdom

Think about the wisdom you learn each day, each year, this lifetime, past lifetimes, and think about how this wisdom influences you to treat others well, how it forms your beliefs, and your actions.

In the six perfections, you have a time-honored tool-box that can bring you to a higher state of consciousness. And through you they can help to change the earth for the better. Developing patience and tolerance allows you to remain calm in a storm and forgo being judgmental. Cultivating concentration and wisdom help you to maintain mental focus on your creativity and learn to not repeat dysfunctional behavior by using the wisdom you gained from past experiences. Practicing joyful effort and generosity helps you learn to develop more of a positive feeling towards work and feel grateful for the rewards that it brings you.

The Nine Deep Healers

In our times, raising consciousness to higher levels needs to include the higher emotional aspects of love. One of the higher aspects of love is being able to forgive others and yourself more easily. Another aspect of love is allowing vulnerability and being slow to anger. Love is also finding contentment and laughter.

It would be very good to devote one week to each group of these deep healers. You should write down all situations that pertain and notice where you fall short and discern what issues you may need to work on. Particularly in being kind to others, notice when you felt compassionate towards others whose suffering was obvious. But beware, because there can be a real pitfall in this. You do not want to get directly involved with them and their suffering because they can and will try to drag you into their circumstances and that would affect you and your own life and undermine your own longevity. I call these attributes the nine deep healers, because once they are mastered, many diseases will vanish.

1. Gratefulness and Appreciation
2. Forgiveness and Apologies
3. Surrender and Vulnerability
4. Kindness, Compassion and Love
5. Higher Consciousness Emotions
6. Contentment and Equanimity
7. Higher Consciousness Thoughts

8. Humor and Laughter
9. Increasing Your Self Worth

For one week pick one of these to work with. You should list the times you worked with each one and you should write down and notice where it was easy for you and where it was hard. This list covers areas that many people have difficulty with.

Gratefulness and Appreciation

Learn to feel gratitude for the things in your life that you appreciate, the large and the small, and for the greatest gift of all, your life. Your body is the most precious thing you own. It allows you to be here.

Forgiveness and Apologies

Many people have difficulty asking for forgiveness and apologizing to others when it is appropriate. Being able to ask for forgiveness and say an apology are important. This is an aspect of deep healing.

Surrender and Vulnerability

Many people have trouble being vulnerable and surrendering to change. They cling to their old habits or fear getting hurt or loosing what they have. Work on surrendering and being vulnerable to change.

Kindness, Compassion and Love

For deep healing, love is the key. Many people tend to block love in their lives. This creates disease. Kindness and compassion are forerunners of love. For one week work on kindness, and compassion, and then love.

Become slow to anger

Anger is a dangerous, damaging emotion that contributes to heart disease. It ages your body, contributes to stress and shortens your life. All conflicts can be resolved peacefully. For one week work on being slow to anger. For one week work to become conscious of when you tend to allow anger and then work on releasing that tendency.

Contentment and Equanimity

Contentment and equanimity are the hallmarks of a master. Contentment means you are contented with what you have, equanimity means you see all people as equal, and this creates peace. These are important traits to work on developing.

Higher Consciousness Thoughts

The higher master numbers have to do with higher consciousness thoughts where you allow only thoughts of higher consciousness. Over time you learn to rid yourself of lower consciousness thoughts and gravitate towards thoughts that basically relate to what is best for all and what is most helpful for the whole group, or city or country or world, where a 'we-ness' replaces today's preoccupation with self.

Humor and Laughter

Laughter is recognized as a hallmark of higher consciousness. Many have difficulties with this, and have been raised to take life too seriously. But laughter is healing. For one week find reasons to laugh.

Increasing Your Self Worth

Low self-worth is one of the biggest problems our civilization faces. Low self-worth creates street people who harbor great anger over their lot in life. Is it our problem? Yes, but not individually—collectively.

Gratefulness and appreciation are steps in allowing you to be kinder and have more compassion and develop the ability to feel and experience and express more love. Asking for forgiveness and being able to apologize are hard to do for many people, but they smooth the energy in any conflict and leave the door open for continued friendship. The inability to surrender to what is best for the whole is at root of many social problems as people want to cling to what they identify with as who they are, and they tend to resist change, and they resist working on attaining higher consciousness and this hinders them and stops their evolutionary process. Vulnerability is an issue with those who have been hurt. But this blocks new relationships and new experiences. Being slow to anger and developing a greater ability to see and use humor and burst into laughter are other important signs of maturity and spiritual development. Developing the ability to be contented, and being able to see others as equal (in that that they all want to be happy) are important steps in being able to cultivate peaceful emotional states. Increasing your sense of self-worth is an on-going assignment for many of us and it involves looking into areas where we not do feel worthy. You are worthy because you were created worthy by God, The Infinite Creator of the All. And moving into a personality where higher consciousness thoughts are practiced on a daily basis is transforming yourself into a higher expression of yourself. When you really master most of these deep healers you will feel more contentment, equanimity and peace. In the six perfections and the nine deep healers, you have two toolboxes that can take you to a higher state of consciousness and put you on the road to life extension.

When you work with these higher consciousness tools you have greater power to adjust your own life cycle. When you can cognize these things, they become you. They can change your life for the better and in this, your current life experience, you can stay here on this planet far beyond your old expected time as you learn how to extend your life. One of the most important things in living a long life is in learning how to love yourself. When you can love yourself, you take care of yourself. This will help you develop the ability to adjust your own life cycle.

Work with these tools because they are part of life extension. Indeed, when you work with the six perfections and the nine deep healers you will accelerate your growth and attain a higher level of consciousness rapidly. Life extension is easier to attain when you are in a higher state of consciousness.

These all are part of attaining perfection. If you can, work with a group when you work with these healing practices. Most people need others around for support. But mastery means you can do it by yourself. Each and every one of you reading this has the potential to become a master. If you can work with these higher consciousness tools by yourself, give yourself a pat on the back, because that means that you are already taking steps to becoming a master.

Love Is the Best Healer of All

As mentioned earlier, I was given a powerful dream that revealed that love can heal. It may help to say it again: "Humans on earth have some damage to their major organs: liver, kidneys, lungs, pancreas, etc., and if humans were able to love each other more, especially with family members, then their own health problems would not be as severe [and they could live longer]. Nutritional healing diets are helpful, but supportive nurturing group are at the root of healing."

Healing: New Energy Healing and Traditional Medical Healing

One of the new emerging concepts about health is that you are born to be healthy and stay healthy all of your life and this will increase more and more as you evolve and as the human civilization evolves. But there will be times when you will need to be healed and the methods below can be used for healing and are important to know. The modes of healing currently available serve humanity and together they represent many methods to restore balance and wellness for the complete range of the human population for all known illness, afflictions and diseases.

The first methods we will talk about are the highest vibration methods available now, and last one is the lowest vibration method, but it is wise not to discard any, because there are some people who will need the lower vibration methods who are not able to relate to the higher vibrational methods. And there are others who have reached a higher consciousness will find that the higher vibration methods will work the best for them.

Energy Healing, Hands on Healing, and Meditation

In energy healing, the energy from the healer so commingles with the client that an energy balance cooperation begins. There is great potential in this that is not yet fully known. This is a non-touch method and it is what the Master from Galilee used. It takes a high vibration healer to use this method. In hands on healing, the individual healer touches the client for healing usually at the afflicted area. Touching makes the bond instead of energy making the bond. This is a wonderful tool and it works, and many healers will be able to do this. Meditation can be a very powerful healing technique that can be developed to a high degree and the individual themself does the healing, although a facilitator may be needed. Several meditation techniques are given in this book that can heal and can slow and even reverse aging to some degree. Meditation techniques should be practiced by the life extension student.

Life Essence Medicines, Colloidal Silver and Magnetics

Live essence medicines were first used to cure tuberculosis and polio. The life force of an imprint does not easily change if the form remains intact. Aroma essence is a form of this. Look for new live essence medicines. Colloidal Silver is a water solution of very small silver ion particles and it is a broad-spectrum anti-pathogen. It is effective against all known pathogens and it is very easy to use and make. Many colloidal silver generators are available on the internet and those that create the small particle size silver ions are very effective. Magnetic healing addresses the magnetic human DNA and it is a valid healing method. There are many healers who place magnets on the body at the proper locations who are healing long standing health problems.

Pharmaceuticals

Medical drugs are a low energy method of healing, yet they should not be discarded because there may be no higher energy methods available for some illnesses. It is important to acknowledge that many lives have been saved by the administration of antibiotics and they will continue have a place because a large percent of the population will continue to strongly relate to them.

Surgery

This is the lowest method and most of the human population has had a surgical operation. Predictions are that this type of healing will be replaced by newer and non-invasive methods, but until they arrive and become established, the wise soul will not dismiss this method if there is no other way to deal with a serious health issue.

Meditation for Healing Any Disease

Along with the new healing and new energy on the planet, there is also the possibility for you to re-program your body to override magnetic imprints from your family's history for some life-threatening disease, and it is also possible for you to rid yourself of a life-threatening disease by speaking out loud the powerful affirmation below. It is important to learn to speak the affirmations out loud but in a low voice when you say any affirmation because doing that sets the energy. Speak out loud to the physical part of your body that you are aware needs healing. Also, speak out loud to the non-physical energy part of your body that you are not aware of that I call your, 'primal energy field', that can help with this healing. And speak out loud all of the cells in your whole body so that they can help with the healing. We will now do this healing meditation affirmation by speaking in a low voice the following words to your whole body, your primal energy, and all of your body's cells. Assume a meditative state, slow your breathing, and become as still as you can.

"My body, and all of the cells in my body, and my primal energy field, hear my instructions. I intend to remove myself from this disease. I give myself permission for this disease to

leave. It is not appropriate. I have much work to do and I cannot let it keep me from doing what I came here to do. And also, it is my intent to not allow my predisposition from my blood line magnetic imprint to express itself."

It is good to start to working in this way. The new healers who use methods like these will be welcomed. The public wants it. With instant communication, thousands will know of the power of the new healing and the floodgates will begin to open to it – to a new healing that is efficient and non-invasive and does not require medications. Imagine a patient or a client reporting to a future healer. Not only will the healer balance the body but disease will ooze out of every cell. It won't have a choice since the body will be receiving instructions on how to eliminate illness. And also, can you imagine looking in the mirror and realizing that you are not aging as much either. Health and balance do that. Next, you will realize that your body didn't only heal, it also received an instruction set from you, the owner. Multidimensional healing is like consciousness homeopathy in which the body receives an instruction set to process things itself. Multidimensional energies speak to the soul, and to the cells, and to the whole body, and to the primal energy field of the individual. A full-body healing doesn't just mean the healing only applies to the organs and mental processes. It also means dealing with the perceptions and traumas from the past. All of this is vital. And all of this is a powerhouse. Indeed, it is and all of this is needed.

Love is the greatest healer of all

Can you open up to a much greater love?
And let that love pour in and be a part of
The new you and then can you send it out?
And open up to greater community without
Your habitual resistance to it and then drop
Your focus on yourself just a little bit – stop
And think about letting a 'we-ness' come in?
If you can do this it will eradicate many sins

And it will rebalance your body into a new
Healthy hemostasis and healing that few
Enjoy and when you send your own love out
It will help heal many others without a doubt.

Your Heart Center is Healing

It is important to learn about your heart center. When you are in your heart center you do not become or take on the anger, pain, and hatred of those who are exuding it that you are trying to resist. You do not want to come into conflict with the good of the world. You need to experience the unity of the world once again and to experience that oneness once again, and the unity and the oneness can be experienced from your heart center. It is not a trivial or insignificant thing to focus on your heart center. You will need to learn to work on staying in your heart center. You can create the world you want by being in your heart center. Here is a meditation to work with your heart center.

Find your heart center now. Enter the front of your heart center which is your heart chakra in your chest. Now move to the back of your heart chakra, and feel the energies as they move into the front and the back of your heart center. Next, do this with your third eye. Move into the front and back of your third eye. Now connect those two, your heart center and your third eye center with a beam of light. Send that beam of light up to the center of the universe and then down into the center of the earth.

Take note of how good that feels and how relaxed you are and how you are able to feel more love. Meditations like this are important for the life extender to begin to add to the repertoire of the life extender's tool box of practices.

Daily Actions of Love

The place of love means the place of community. It is important to work with love on a daily basis. It is important to put more love in your heart. We as a civilization, although local wars will still happen for a while, are beginning to create the new earth. In a very real sense, it appears that we are accomplishing the impossible.

Can you believe that lack of love causes disease? It does. It would be a giant step forward for you to be able to hold love in your heart and mind and send it out to others and to yourself continually, every day from this day forward. But you will find that your thoughts will dip back into negative lower worlds. When this happens, don't let other such thoughts follow. Say, "Cancel," and then refocus on love and say the word, "Love…" seven times, "love, love, love, love, love, love, love". Over time this technique will help to sweep negative thoughts from your mind. Your mind, which unfortunately has habituated lower thoughts from the old energy will slowly begin to say, "I accept that this is not me, and then the words 'cancel' and 'love' will erase many of the negative thoughts from your mind and your mind will again begin to find a living peace. It is important to go about your day in a world that you can feel internally as inner peace that you exist within. Now, as you do your chores and as you wash the dishes, send love to the water which will join with the river and ocean and a healing of the waters might occur. As you brush your teeth and shower don't fret about your day, but instead make an intention to focus on the cleansing, healing and rejuvenating affect that the shower does for every cell in your body. As you go about your day thing about the healing and regenerating that your deeper breathing does. It is a good idea to get into the habit of doing this. Every time you shower, make an intention that the water running over your skin not only cleanses your body but also rejuvenates it and removes the aetheric toxins that are placed there for that very purpose. Every time you do breathwork make an intention that it adds oxygen and prana that you can use for healing and regeneration. Every time you do fasting make an intention that it cleanses and breaks down and removes old and worm out senescent cells. It is in making these small intentions in your daily activities that creates a huge difference in your daily reality.

At breakfast, be thankful for the food and run your hand over it and say to yourself, "this is healthy food for me." It is the agreement you have with the food that is most important. In time your body will tell you what is best to eat and drink. When you greet family members use a hug or an imaginary hug. When you drive to and from work, don't fight and fret about the traffic, for it is well known to lower your vibration. Instead, redirect your thoughts to your breathing and slowly think of the things you love. Before you enter work, pause a moment and breathe into it and then count from 1 to 10 and enter as if you were the best employee ever. Let your mind, body and soul merge and become one. If your day gets away from you (as it will from time to time) and you drop in vibration, reconnect to your heart. And as you leave work fill it with light and know that this thought will change the vibration for tomorrow. When you acknowledge the times, you have been brought down by others, say, "release, release, release." Or if it is a particular low vibration, you can call upon higher beings for help. On the way home if you stop at a grocery store, send love to all in the store and infuse all food with love and health. At night as you are going to bed be thankful for the good things that happened during the day. And intend that the extra oxygen and prana from your breathing practices be used for tissue repair, enhanced cellular regeneration, and life extension. And when you are fasting intend that the purification and removal of old cells be used for life extension. Choose how you live, but put love and intention into your day every day.

A Deep Healing Meditation

Many healers have used meditation to heal the sick and severely traumatized. They instruct their clients to let go of their trauma and just let their conscious go to their perfect place of peace, which might be a church, or a sanctuary, or the beach, at the ocean, or it might even be in the great void. Slowly but surely, little by little, the client's health is usually gradually restored. As the client's health improves, medications can be reduced, and over time complete recovery is often reported. There are many case histories that strongly demonstrate that when the underlying emotional trauma ruminations are stopped, the body can and will return back into its natural, normal state of balance and health. To heal severe trauma and injury, this meditation technique will need to be performed many times over a long period time – it may take an hour a day for perhaps several months to heal a severe life-threatening injury and debilitating trauma.

Assume your meditation position, calm your breathing, and become as still as you can. Go into your place of perfect peace. It could be a church, a sanctuary, an ocean beach, or even the great void. Begin to know that you are in a place where you are not concerned about time. Allow your mind to dissolve into the idea of space and no form until you feel the nothingness, the nothing at all but you and your consciousness and the peacefulness. Feal the peace that is all around you in your place of perfect peace. Bask in this peace. Do not allow any thoughts about any trauma or any distraction invade your mind. If they come, return to that place of perfect peace or the great void and return to the peace that you feel there. Do not let that peace become interrupted or disturbed. Let yourself bask in this peace and feel that your health issue is slowly being brought back into its balanced, normal, and healed state.

DNA, Stem Cell Healing

It is important to note that the DNA in each and every cell in your body is connected to all of the other millions of DNA in all of the other millions of cells of your body though an energy field that I call your 'Primal Energy Field.' This field has also been called: 'the innate,' or 'the merkabah,' or 'the auric field' or even 'the energy body.' At the quantum atomic level, it is a multidimensional field that connects all of your DNA together, and it has one intelligence, and most importantly, it is connected to your original body template or blueprint. That means that it knows how your body should be as compared to your original body blueprint. It also means that it knows what a human wants and needs, and when a human gives instruction for the body to heal, it knows like homeopathy 'knows' exactly what the human is trying to heal and it is benevolent to the upmost.

You have the opportunity to heal yourself of any condition by giving instructions combined with powerful intention. First, you need to use conceptualized thought. Next, you need to see and visualized yourself being healed. And last, you need to see yourself out of your disease or infirmity. These are the instruction sets that you will need to be giving that will go right into your DNA that has receptors that are far more willing and ready to receive your information then you ever thought or realized or knew existed. The cures can be simple and quick. But the realignment and facilitation of the new energies will take some time so you will need to allow for that. When you work with healing through your primal energy field this offers a powerful increase in healing because it is working with the body intelligence in your primal energy field which is quantum at the atomic level and is quite benevolent. When you do a DNA quantum stem cell healing meditation, the more refined your instructions are, the more benevolence is seen and understood by your body and it will start to heal through your master template. Your master template (which is the basic blueprint of your body) is stored in your DNA and is connected to your primal energy field. And your master template has received an upgrade recently to the newer more evolved human.

All of the DNA of your body is singular having only one allied consciousness and it is quantumly locked together so that it works as one benevolent union, and it connects to your smart body which I call your 'primal energy field' body. This energy field around your DNA is quantum and its response is not linear, not chemical, and not intellectual. At the quantum level, this multidimensional field that connects all of your DNA together has one intelligence, and it is connected to your original body template, the original blueprint of your body (now upgraded) and that is important. This means that it knows exactly what you are trying to do. It is important to emphasize that in working with healing in this way that you begin to bring in the higher consciousness attributes of compassion, tolerance, temperance, generosity, kindness and gratitude. Also, you should begin to bring in what I call your spirit team. Your spirit team is your spirit guides, the ascended masters and the angles and archangels. So, now let us do a DNA, quantum stem cell healing. But before we start google stem cell and memorize what it looks like.

Assume your meditative state, become very calm, very relaxed, and very, very still. Feel the energies of compassion, tolerance, temperance, generosity, kindness and gratitude flow into your heart, and now ask for your spirit team (your spirit guides, the ascended masters, and the angles and the archangels) to be with you and help you. Next, intuitively visualize the area of your body that needs healing. Now visualize just one of your stem cells (and remember stem cells are in every cell and they are all quantumly connected to each other and to your primal energy field so that many more of them will benevolently join in). And now, speak out loud to the DNA of your body's cells that need to be healed and say, "beloved cells, I am your boss, your owner, and I instruct your healing to proceed." Now visualize just that one stem cell. Be specific and speak out loud to that one stem cell and say, "Dear stem cell, I want the visualized area of my body healed, and I ask that you go to the visualized area of my body that needs to be healed and stay there and begin to replicate new tissue there right now!" And then intuit that your healing is beginning to happen. Believe that it is unfolding, and let it happen.

Other Types of Healing for Your Physical Body

There are many hot springs around the world, and they are traditionally acknowledged as healing centers for the healing they can bring in their hot water soak pools. Some have a cold-water pool nearby and this combination is an exceptionally strong ancient healing practice because it creates what is known as the 'hot-cold shock' effect which sends the body into a deep healing overdrive. There are radon health spas and radon health mines worldwide and many cures from very difficult health issues have been reported with radon. Colon hydrotherapy treatments are said to be able to remove plaque from the arteries. Lite water has reported anti-cancer properties, especially when injected directly into a tumor. Many herbs and herbal combinations have strong healing properties. Cures have been reported from breath work practices, and mastery of some of the many breath cycles can heal, extend your life and keep you younger. Fasting is healing. There are many reports of cures of health conditions from fasting, especially with fasts in the intermediate range of two to four weeks. And colloidal silver is good at curbing, and in many cases curing, infectious diseases of all kinds. Exercise and yoga stretching are actually healing. The body needs to be used and kept flexible and it needs some physical exercise and stretching.

Healing for your Soul

Many people have a soul trait that is an out of balance condition within their soul. The overly aggressive and excessively meek personality traits are two of them. These need to be corrected. How do you heal an imbalance of the soul such as the overly aggressively trait or the too meek trait? Well, first, you have to recognize it and acknowledge that it exists and then begin to become aware of this negative trait whenever it shows up and surfaces, such as the when the over aggressive soul trait asserts itself by taking an overly aggressively stance on some issue, or when the too meek soul trait asserts itself by being overly meek in situations where this is inappropriate. Then through grace, and through asking for help, intend that this imbalance within the soul be transformed into a milder version of the negative trait.

Psychiatry for Aberrant Mental Health

Severe mental and emotional health issues will hinder your spiritual growth and take a toll on your longevity. These need to treated. For those with severe aberrant behavior tendencies and traits, the benefits from being treated by a psychiatrist or clinical mental health staff cannot be overstated. Correcting aberrant traits of the personality complex is very important. It is a good idea to become familiar with typical neurotic behavior types and abnormal personality traits by reading up on this in lay psychiatric literature.

There Is a Higher Purpose for Disease

As the human race evolves, people may eventually come to accept that there is always a higher purpose for disease. A most important purpose. A purpose that goes unrecognized by the human race at the present time. There are a few with higher consciousness who know the purpose for disease and as such they do not fear disease because they know that after it has run its course and completed its cycle they will feel better afterwards because of the deep cleansing that the bacteria or virus infection does when it breaks down tissue and releases toxins even some deeply seated toxins. The location in the body is always symbolic and it reflects the issues going on in your life. The higher purpose is always linked to the law of symbols so that through the symbolic reflection that the disease brings, some effort can be made to correct the issue. For example, a severe cold has respiratory symptoms (runny nose, coughing, sore throat and chest congestion) and these all symbolize a strong negative emotional issue connected with speech (because the lungs propel the air to make the speech). And so, the higher purpose for a bad cold may well be to work with higher consciousness and wisdom from similar prior events and learn to not allow the emotions to run amuck and get whipped up into a negative frenzy over some negative life situation and just accept what is with serenity.

Those Who Know This Do Not Fear Disease

Indeed, they do not fear disease and they may even come to welcome it. They know that disease offers a cleansing and purification opportunity. They are skilled healers and they know that their body will overcome any disease and they look forward to the cleansing that the disease will bring. They also understand such things as the underlying causes of epidemics. If, for example, a bird flu epidemic were to break out, they know that birds are symbolic of freedom (since birds with their flight have the most freedom of all the animals) and they would immediately connect the bird flu outbreak with some restriction of freedom for the humans who live in the area of the outbreak.

It would be a good idea for the life extension student to begin to understand and work with the higher purpose for disease and then eventually come to not fear any disease. All of the healing methods should be used, of course, with any disease, but one need not fear disease as such.

Activating the 24th Chromosome Pair

We will now launch into a more advanced healing modality, which involves activating the 24th chromosome pair. Humans have 23 chromosome pairs that science can see and knows about, but there is actually a 24th pair that science cannot see and does not know about because it is interdimensional. But before we start, we will give a short preamble about why activating the 24th Chromosome pair is necessary now. We will say that before humans can activate the 24th chromosome pair they will first need to learn how to tap into the multidimensional realities and into the bigger soul group. This is because it is important to remember the wisdom from the past and you can do this when you develop the ability to access your multidimensional realities. Much longer life times are necessary now because if human have to start over again every single time they are born, they will not be able to access the wisdom from the past and that is one of the important reasons why increased longevity is so necessary. It is necessary so that the whole human group has the wisdom from the past to finally and fully understand that war never works. It is absolutely necessary for the human group to learn this truth. How many generations will it take? What if you did not have to be born again and again? In the future the world will be far more benevolent and multidimensional than it is now.

You do have a 24th chromosome pair that is latent now and not yet active, but it will become active, and when it does you will start having multidimensional biology which might be called a super smart primal energy field because it will be so smart that it will never allow disease to invade it. It will be smarter than the old diseases. Your biological defense system won't let disease come in. What do you think this might do to your longevity and how long humans are supposed to live? Consider this – no more Alzheimer's, no more cancer – all diseases will be seen as dysfunctional and stupid to an evolved human that has a super active 24th chromosome pair. Your immune defense will become a super defense. Multidimensional biology is smart – so smart that disease cannot invade it, because it is smarter than the old energy diseases of the earth. It will be like medical science of yesteryear giving the body a tincture of what to look for (like the flu shots of today) so that the body would know what to look for and wouldn't let it in. In the future when the 24th chromosome pair is fully activated, an idea of this will be that the body itself will make this tincture and thus it will not let the disease in. This will completely change expectations about how long a human can live when the body can eliminate cancer and dementia and all the other diseases in this way. Name any disease that is common today and after the 24th chromosome pair becomes activated, the disease will not be allowed in that body because the immune defense system of the light body will become a super immune defense, and as this happens, human lifespans will literally skyrocket! Let us do a meditation now to begin to activate to some extent your 24th chromosome pair. Before doing this meditation, if would be smart to google 'chromosome' to get a good idea of what they look like.

Become calm and still and bring in your spirit guide team (your guides, the ascended masters and the angles) and your primal energy field. Direct your mind to image one of your present 23 chromosome pairs, and then intend to see your interdimensional 24th chromosome pair. Just let whatever image comes up linger for a while and then speak in a low voice to your primal energy field and to your spirit guide team and say, "I ask that my latent 24th chromosome pair begin to become active and begin to become a multidimensional biology which might be called a super smart primal energy field that is so smart that it will start making a 'tincture' of what to look for (like today's flu shots) for any invading bacteria or virus so that my body will develop antibodies on its own that will disable the invading disease pathogen." Speak again, "I ask that my 24th chromosome pair become activated to the degree that my light quotient allows and connected to my multidimensional biology's primal energy field that is so smart that it will not let disease in and this will allow my life span to really soar."

Now begin to intuit this happening, and know that to some degree it will begin to happen. Then say, "thank you," to your spirit guide team and your primal energy field.

Your Body Is Always Healthy

Your body is always healthy. Your body is always healthy and whole. It is your beliefs about your body that cause it to be not healthy and not whole. It is your responsibility to remember that your body is a gift and not something to let go of. It is your responsibility to remember that the normal state of your body is health. It is your responsibility to know it and to accept it as a given.

Chants for health and longevity

Let us sing a few chants for health and longevity now. And when you sing these chants be playful about it. You don't have to be super serious about this life extension business, you know. You can be playful with it. You can have fun with it. You can enjoy working with it. Repeat each chant several times.

My body is in good health as all the world can see.
I never worry about disease – no disease for me!

My body is my servant and I love to make it stronger.
My body's cells are healthy and they want to live longer.

Do you want to live longer?

Then develop higher consciousness by working with the six perfections and the nine deep healers. Get into the habit of keeping your heart center open. Do the needed affirmations and meditations and chants often and do them one chapter at a time. Pick at least one life extension affirmation to say every morning as soon as you wake up and get out of bed and then say it in a low voice. Let the words of the affirmation sink in.

Do this every morning. I dare you! Do you want to live longer? Then do the work in each chapter many times! When you do this, you are going to feel it happening. And you will find that it will happen. It's like exercising energy – the more you hear it and the more you say it, and the more you do it, the more your neurons fire and come together to create it, do you understand this? When you cognize things, they become you. It's a circle and it starts with you saying your affirmations and doing your meditations and it's never been more powerful then now!

The masters were able to live without disease and they said, "What I can do, you can [learn] to do also."

CHAPTER 5
Higher Consciousness

Cultivate the red rose of compassion and let it bloom.
Daily nurture its soil and send it never ending kindness.
Tenderly water it with equanimity so as to give it room.
For the cool shade of joy so that it knows it is blessed.

Life extension students in our times need to be taught somewhat different purification practices that lean more towards attaining higher consciousness levels. Indeed, life extension is a natural result of developing the skills of the six perfections as taught in Buddhist's monasteries, and the nine deep healers that I am introducing. And attaining higher consciousness also involves learning about the twelve universal laws of creation. When you really begin to accept this and learn them such that they become incorporated into your own personality complex, you begin to realize that many illnesses that could have come to you are nipped in the bud. Not only does attaining a higher consciousness level lead to a longer life span and absence of disease, but it also brings a sense of contentment, equanimity and peace. The ancient physical immortality practices of mastering the mind's thought patterns, and mastering the emotional states for attaining a state of contentment, of course, still apply, but we will work with them now in a more modern setting.

The Sub-Human State
Alchemy was a forerunner of today's requirement that humanity transform itself from the gross state of survival

at any cost which usually involves forced conflict, into a higher spiritual consciousness where all are valued and where forced conflict is abhorred. And the process of evolving consciousness requires continual refinement. In the beginning, we learn to curb violence by refraining from harming or killing others. But as consciousness matures, we realize that it is indeed an act of violence to 'harm or kill' another's joy, happiness or peace of mind. Moving into higher and higher levels, one learns to contain, maintain, and generate the highest frequencies and that is a skill to be very grateful for.

Sri Aurobindo was a brilliant futurist from India, and he contemplated human development and was able to notice that human consciousness has a number of levels or states of evolutionary growth. The beginning level he termed the sub-human level. And then he outlined a number of higher levels of ascending consciousness as humans evolve in spiritual development. It is important to understand this at his sub-human state because that is the level that a large percent of unevolved humans still exist at.

His sub-human referred to the humans of today who have not evolved at all spiritually. His insight was brilliant and he noticed and intuited the connection of his sub-human state to the plant and animal kingdoms. Although far from being connected to them physically they still continue to be connected to them in their level of consciousness. His sub-human state is characterized by people clinging to their own 'roots', being quick to 'vegetate', and tending to have subconscious animalistic 'nomadic and predatory habits', as well as a 'blind servility' to the custom and 'rule of the pack'. Among these animalist qualities that Aurobindo called sub-human were tendencies toward mob behavior mentality and lower psychic abilities and communication, and where most people were utterly open to input from the mass mentality and the mass collective subconsciousness. He also found that most sub-human people tend to be dominated by rage and fear much like in animal behavior. He also saw that most of those people were actually afraid of and incapable of accepting and living in true freedom. He realized that this is a basic attribute of the sub-human state.

He also noticed that in this unenlightened state that most people harbored a great distrust of anything new as well as demonstrating a difficulty in grasping and assimilating new ideas with the quickness of those who have achieved a higher state of consciousness. He observed that the propensity that most people have for heaviness is revealed by the downward gazes that they have. He also connected humanity's subjection to heredity as an animalistic trait.

Aurobindo's lowest level of consciousness, the sub-human level, is basically the level of mankind before 2012, and it is now slowly raising. As it raises, it exchanges those animalistic and plant traits for progressively greater and greater states of enlightened consciousness. It is interesting to look at his further insights by reflecting on mankind's 'unconscious servitude to custom' as well as its homage to 'pack mentality' that could be the driving forces behind today's rampant divisiveness and intolerance that leads to deep schisms which erupt into forceful conflicts and warfare around the globe. At higher states of consciousness, one learns to generate the wisdom to contain and direct the highest frequencies of pure consciousness by being able see the whole world as yourself and seeing an energetic blanket of love and peace enfolding the earth.

Cultivating Compassion

Cultivating compassion is indeed the main road to higher consciousness and also plays an important role in attaining life extension. Compassion is at the root of developing higher consciousness, and higher consciousness is needed for your DNA to work at a higher efficiency level then the 35% that it is working at now and this is one of the keys to life extension. Teaching the cultivation of compassion has always been a major training in many of the traditional schools of enlightenment, especially among the Buddhist's. Indeed, the Buddha's teachings all revolve around compassion. And it turns out that meditating on compassion is actually a very good way to achieve a state of compassion.

Many people will agree that compassion or having and feeling empathy for others who are suffering is represented by some act of kindness. Kindness is connected to compassion. Here is an interesting example of the power of kindness. A man wanted to make the world a kinder place. A yoga master suggested to him that whenever he met a person coming toward him to look into the face of that one and offer a smile. By doing this only a few times he learned that one person could, in fact, make a difference in a very large world. He was amazed to notice now many people who were walking very heavy hearted actually responded to his smile by returning one. In the briefest of exchanges such as this he was able to communicate warmth and even a field of harmony. If genuine, a simple smile can offer loving kindness and very important, it can engender a state of equanimity in the one who offers the smile.

In spiritual practices generating compassion begins with meditating on equanimity. And this in turn leads to developing a capacity to hold a mental state of impartiality, or neutrality, towards one's self and towards all others. In a deeper sense, in a greater understanding, this involves eliminating attachments and aversion so that you let a kind of neutrality rise. This neutrality is what the man offered when he smiled at a complete stranger. He could simply meet the other, send loving energy through a smile, and then in passing, wish the other person well and it turns out that this is a basic form of the Buddha Bodhicitta practice.

In every aspect of your life there are those men and women that you hold dear, those that you have an aversion towards. and those that you are neutral towards. To really experience true neutrality, you must learn to see all sentient life as equal and this includes people, animals, and even insects. When we carefully analyze this, it reveals that the kind of feelings you have for those you hold dear are based on attachments, and the feelings you have for those you hold as evil are based on a negative experience with them. When we look deeper into both the positive and the negative feelings we have for others, we find that in most cases the behaviors that both groups offer that we have positive feelings about or negative feelings about comes mainly from the kinds of life circumstance that they have experienced. And when it comes to actually cultivating compassion, meditation approaches offer important benefits and leads to higher consciousness.

Before starting the meditation, carefully consider the uncertainty of all relationships. Friends and lovers may part or die. The suffering from disagreement, anger, or hostility can erupt even in the closest of relationships. And all relationships must be seen as transitory. We will begin by choosing three relationships and then expand it to include all potential relationships. For the three relationships chose someone you are completely neutral towards – perhaps someone in a store you shop at but know nothing about, and then choose someone who is a friend or one you have benefited from, and then choose someone you harbor anger towards due to having been harmed by them. Next, choose people at large – a politician, a street person, a coworker, a warfighter in combat, a dentist, and perhaps someone in the news who is in a difficult position. Then carefully notice how your mind reacts to each of them.

Meditation for Cultivating Compassion -1st part

Become calm, and still, and go into meditation and bring in your spirit guide team. Now bring into your mental screen in succession, a friend you have benefited from, someone you are neutral about, and a person that you are at odds with. Bring them in one at a time and watch how your mind reacts to each of them. When you see the friend, your mind is calm and peaceful (it may even want to remember pleasant moments with them, but resist this and just notice the state of your mind). With your foe, your mind may become agitated, irritated or resentful. But, with the stranger, your mind has no stories or reactions to cling to – there is no delight, disgust or annoyance, only neutrality. Now bring into your mental screen the others, one at a time: the poor, the rich, the educated, the illiterate, those in high station, and ordinary people. Notice how your mind reacts to each of them.

Notice that your mental states for each of them derives from attitudes that are quite superficial and self-serving. For your friend your mental state of calmness comes from attachments to benefits derived from them, but for your foe your mental state of agitation comes from past unpleasant experiences with them. It is only with the stranger that your mental states are neutral because you have no experience with them either pleasant or unpleasant. For the poor your mental state might be aversion; for the rich, envy; for the educated, acceptance; and for the illiterate, rejection. Begin to accept that your mind reacts to different people because of your feelings about your own past experiences with them (for those you know), and by your conditioned attitude about the kind of lives they lead (for those you don't know), and by your many past lives.

Meditation for Cultivating Compassion -2nd part

Now, go back in meditation and begin to see the suffering in each of them. The rich suffer because they fear losing their wealth, the poor suffer because of their lack, and the others suffer because of their own areas of discontentment and disappointment. As they appear on your mental screen, carefully note that in terms of desiring happiness, they are all equal. They all want to be free from their respective types of suffering, and in that, they are all the same. Let the suffering of all beings be shown to you. As they appear on your mental screen, carefully note that in terms of desiring happiness, they are all equal. They all want to be free from their respective types of suffering, and in that, they are all the same. As you observe them one by one carefully reflect on the suffering of all beings. Carefully reflect on the area of suffering of each person on your mental screen. Let your heart be moved by seeing their suffering, and let your mind keep reminding you that they only want to be happy.

Next include yourself. Look compassionately at your own areas of discontentment and disappointment and simply acknowledge that all beings suffer in one way or another. Allow yourself to begin to feel and see this deeply. You will start to experience profound compassion. It will also become quite apparent to you that all beings are profoundly connected to one another. And you will know that it is quite literally true that the happiness or suffering of one person directly affects the whole. All consciousness in the universe is utterly and unequivocally interconnected—and this is really the Universal Law of Love. Let yourself know that this mutual dependency that flows human to human generates a collective web of experiencing.

When practiced over time, this contemplative technique can lead you into a mental state of impartiality toward all beings, including pets, other animals and all wildlife and even insects. No matter how many faces you visualize, all want exactly the same outcome when it comes to achieving happiness and avoiding suffering. If practiced over time this contemplative technique can lead you into a mental state of impartiality toward all beings including pets, other animals and all wildlife and even insects.

This meditation has been used by Buddhas-in-training for many thousands of years. When practiced regularly, it will open the awakening mind to bodhicitta or profound compassion. As you learn equanimity (to see them all as equal) toward all created beings you will quite naturally develop a precious closeness to them. The fruits of love will increase and the more you find all life important, the more you will be concerned about their suffering. And meditations on equanimity thus naturally evolve into reflections of loving kindness and love. The life extension student should work on this meditation with the goal of striving for a state of equanimity, to see everyone as equal in wanting to avoid suffering. Then you should begin to feel their suffering and struggle; individually at first, and then in groups, nations, and then the whole world. You should work on it until you really know that you have truly developed compassion, and when it becomes fully developed, tears may start to come to your eyes when you see a situation that creates great suffering that invokes a strong feeling of compassion in you. Compassion is a foundation for life extension!

Compassion Replaces 'I' with 'We' Consciousness

Let us consider what changes in the mind in the process of its emancipation, and let us ask from what is the mind liberated from? In the process of attaining enlightenment, both the mind and the notion of the "I" changes radically. The mind expands to gradually allow higher resonant frequencies of enlightenment to be explored, realized, and ultimately embodied, and then the preoccupation with the 'I' begins to fade. Concerns for your own welfare gradually become replaced with concerns for the welfare of others. And then your mind will expand and your own problems will seem smaller, less demanding and easier to face. In the end, believe it or not, the real beneficiary of compassion is you. The practice of compassion builds inner strength and bestows inner peace.

Sri Aurobindo's Ladder of Evolving Consciousness

Aurobindo's analysis in his written works were divinely inspired and negotiating his ladder of ascending consciousness involves awakenings all along the way. He noted that spiritual development and maturation are based on a life of service. He saw life itself as a gracious act of service. Stated another way, your life is not totally about you, but unfortunately many have much resistance to making this shift in consciousness. Here is a very brief synopsis of Sri Aurobindo's ladder of evolving consciousness.

<u>Sub Human</u> – lowest level, has major animalistic traits – survival and domination over others
<u>Higher Mind</u> – connection and mental clarity to spirit, beginning compassion, desire to live longer
<u>Illuminated Mind</u> – Striking clarity, compassionate thought is at the root of the luminous mind
<u>Intuitive Mind</u> – Nurturing the wisdom that realizes the true, or empty nature of everything

<u>Cosmic Consciousnesses</u> – Inner presence of spiritual light, universe is a consciousness permeating all
<u>Super mind</u> – the level at which direct union with the Creative Source can be consummated.

To climb Aurobindo's ladder, you must train the mind to bring this about – you must cultivate the three attributes of enlightenment. But all of these are simply various manifestations of compassion. And in a nutshell, all of the Buddha's teaching centers around cultivating compassion. The plethora of world material manifestations are simply seen as tools of spirit. At the super mind stage, physical perfection can be fully realized. In Aurobindo's teaching, this upward movement is met, complimented, and enhanced by a concurrent downward descending flow from the higher self or soul. The upward flow is utterly dependent on the downward flow. Aurobindo's analysis is both sophisticated and divinely inspired and negotiating his ladder of ascending consciousness involves awakenings all along the way.

Meditating on compassion is a good first passive approach, but sending compassion and love to war torn areas, to the homeless, to the sick, to all who are suffering in one way or another, is a more in-depth active approach and it is what future humans on earth will do. In spiritual practice generating compassion by meditating on equanimity is cultivating the mind set of holding mental states of impartiality and neutrality towards all others no matter what their status in life is, whether rich or poor, whether CEO or homeless, whether healthy or sick. As one works to remove mental states of attachment which creates fondness for friends and aversion or repulsion for foes, eventually a state of neutrality emerges. To experience true equanimity, you must expand this to include all sentient beings, all lifeforms on the planet: plants, animals, even insects. You will need to reflect on the suffering of all beings: the animal that might starve in the winter, the plant that has not enough water in the summer, the human who has acquired more material possessions then most yet who is still unhappy because he feels he should have even more or that someone might take what he has. All suffer – even the kings of yesteryear suffered!

More on Cultivating Compassion

Your own spiritual growth development depends on your growing dedication to putting an end to suffering of all types including forced conflict and even all warfare. Attaining the omniscient mind is through this route. Supreme enlightenment is simply an on-going practice of entering a mind state of truly wishing that all beings find a way to experience ongoing happiness. To experience true equanimity, you must learn to see all sentient beings equally. This means to detach from attachments and aversions. This means to reflect on the suffering of all beings. Eventually the mind's parched landscape is watered with the gentle rain of loving kindness and the seeds of compassion once planted will take root and grow and burst forward into glorious blooms of love. And that includes people, animals and even insects.

Liberate Yourself from Powerful Kleshas

Klesha is a Sanskrit word that translates as an afflictive mental state and the three of these that are most often mentioned are: greed, hatred, and delusion. Greed manifests as reaching, wanting, grasping, and holding something that you think you need—consumerism is greed based. Greed is basically attachment. Hatred is attempting to push away what is not wanted. Indeed, both greed and hatred can arouse inner states of aversion. Hatred shows up in stubbornness, anger, quarrelsomeness, and aversion. Delusion is a false mental state of entertaining superiority, and ego aggrandizement, and also states of inferiority and hopelessness. Personal delusion includes states of: confusion, ambivalence, indecisiveness, laziness, self-preoccupation, deceit, self-doubt, general ineptitude, self-pity and even avoiding responsibility. To realize the enlightened state, it is important to root out all of these kleshas that will block your growth.

Resisting Buddha Consciousness

Humanity by and large tends to resist Buddha consciousness. It is a struggle to attain enlightenment. Buddha says that suffering is evident to the degree that one experiences discontentment. St. Paul, even when he was in prison was able to write his remarkable, 'choosing to be content,' statement to his followers: "For I have learned that in whatever state I am in therewith to be content." Even today spiritual aspirants are instructed to accept whatever life offers and rather than resist arising circumstances and conditions, to learn from them and remain content with them. One of Buddha's greatest offerings was in revealing the cause of afflictive mental states. He taught extensively the forces of the mind that prevent the experience of contentment. The forces that obscure the goal of contentment are basically because people today get caught up in greed, aversion or mental delusion – the three Kleshas. It is these states of the mind that must be transcended to reach enlightenment.

The Twelve Universal Laws and Higher Consciousness

Another aspect of higher consciousness is to learn and work with the twelve universal creative principles usually called 'The Twelve Universal Laws,' that the Supreme Creator gave to its creation. Each of these principles or laws is an aspect of creation itself. And to understand them is to understand creation. And in each of these universal laws there is an aspect of longevity and life extension. And so, it is important, even imperative, to begin to learn and work with these twelve creative principles for developing higher consciousness and to add them to your life extension knowledge base.

The Universal Law of Manifestation

The law of manifestation says that the sole reason for form of any kind is for spirit to indwell in it, to use it as a home, a vehicle, a body to use and live within, to have experience, and eventually come to know itself, or to come to self-realization. Therefore, all form has spirit within it, from the simplest stones; to the trees, shrubs, grasses; to the birds, insects, humans; and to the moons, planets, stars and galaxies. This is the most important of the Creator's universal laws because without it there would be no created universe and no life forms to experience the creation.

The Universal Law of Thought

The law of thought says, "Thought is the creative force of the universe." What you think about with strong emotion is what you create. Humans tend to use thought in negative ways regarding health issues. When humans think about some worrisome health issue, they become powerfully involved in actually creating it. When they think positive thoughts about getting a job, or a relationship, they manifest it. A higher knowledge of thought patterns is to understand that they can create thought-forms, and these thought-forms are created entities unto themselves and they attach to their originator and they tend to impulse their originator to carry out the intent of the thought, and that is why negative thoughts are so dangerous. As humans evolve, direct mind-to-mind telepathic communication begins. Humans who are evolving to higher consciousness levels will need to learn to begin to control their thoughts such that they are positive and reflect ideas that are for the benefit of all.

The Universal Law of Speech

The law of speech says, "Speech will be used to influence." Every life form in the universe speaks: bacteria speak, as do plants, animals, humans, ascended masters, non-physical entities, moons, stars, star clusters, and galaxies. Speech can be, of course, constructive or destructive, and helpful or hurtful. Much critical, condemning speech is meted out daily by the human group and this causes heavy karma. Speech can come from the past, the present or the future, and you can send it to the past, present or future. Some people can hear plants speak. Animals speak both through vocal means and through telepathy. Ascended masters and other non-physical beings speak though telepathic sound, or blocks of thought. For humans who are evolving into higher consciousness, speech is carefully used with carefully chosen words to influence in kind, helpful, benevolent and compassionate ideas.

The Universal Law of Reflection

The law of reflection is often stated as, "As above, so below; as within, so without." By the law of reflection, we know that the spirit that dwells within a rock has progressed far less in its evolutionary journey cycles than the spirit that dwells within a plant or an animal or a human. By reflection, any sickness reflects an out-of-balance condition with symbols that identify the nature of the out-of-balance state. How you relate to and react to others, how you go about your day, whether your day is a good day or a bad day, whether you have plenty or suffer lack, are all direct reflections of your personality consciousness within. To some extend the microcosm may be a reflection of the macrocosm.

The Universal Law of Symbols

The law of symbols says, "Symbols in which one thing will stand for another will be used for teaching life lessons." Symbols are everywhere. The oval outline of a tree is a symbol that says these trees bear fruit to sustain life that comes from the oval shaped womb. The steeple shaped trees of the forest are symbols that reflect the reverence that the forest provides. The law of symbols comes into play in human health issues. There is a symbol in the body part affected in all illness. For dementia, the symbol of the afflicted mind reflects a lopsided overuse of the mind in the three-sided triangle of beingness: the physical, the emotional, and the mental. Many dementia sufferers overuse the mind by continually speaking out about their unhappiness and not getting much out of life, and they suppress the other two sides of their being – their physical and emotional sides. For heart disease sufferers it is clear that the symbol of the heart – love of self and others, reflects to them an out-of-balanced state regarding their own lack of self-love, often in a smoking addiction and a driving personality to accomplish regardless of the consequences. For diabetics, the symbol of the failed pancreas (that body part that processes sweet foodstuffs) reflects the fact that the life in progress has failed to allow adequate sweetness to keep the body fit and to enjoy a sweet lifestyle. Diabetics frequently tend to substitute sweet pastries for sweet relationships and an enjoyable (sweet) lifestyle.

The Universal Law of Permanence

The law of permanence has to do with the level or degree of integration of the spirit that indwells a form. For the higher animals and humans, the spirit complex is integrated enough that the spirit-soul stays together as a single spirit entity upon the demise of its physical host vehicle. For all animal forms lower than bees, and for the entire plant kingdom, the spirit that indwells them is not integrated enough to maintain itself as a singular entity, and when the host physical form dies, the spirit in it goes to a group collective spirit of the animal or plant at the level attained. The degree of integration of the spirit in any form is also linked to the permanence of the physical vehicle it occupies – the greater the integration of the spirit with the Source is, the more permanent the physical vehicle and the longer the potential lifespan can last. But the greater the separation from Source, the less permanent the physical vehicle generally. The spirit complex of a planet or a star is very integrated and planets and stars can last for millions of years. Permanence is also linked to the idea of the I AM, especially as it relates to the I AM a spark of the Creator God.

The Universal Law of Progression

The law of progression says that there is no stagnation in the universe in which things never change, there is only movement to the next phase of a cycle. Colloquially – the only constant in the universe is change. The law of progression is the reason why chronic diseases always progressively get worse unless the body condition is brought back into a hemostasis balance. All spirit has a natural progression to evolve and graduate to the next phase of its evolutionary cycle. The usual progression of spirit is to progress through the five stages of development starting with the kingdom of the air, then graduating to the mineral kingdom, then the kingdom of the plants, then the animals and finally the humans. Each of these phases can last a cosmic day. A cosmic day may last millions of years. In each phase, there are lessons that the spirit must learn. For the air and mineral kingdoms, it is to learn and assimilate the home planet's vibrations; for the plant phase, to provide oxygen and food for the animals and humans; for the animal phase, to learn the lesson of survival; and for the human phase to evolve in consciousness spiritually and technologically.

The Universal Law of Cycles

The law of cycles says there is a cycle to everything in the universe. There is the daily cycle of night and day; there is the yearly cycle of the seasons: spring, summer, autumn, and winter; there is the life cycle of plants, animals and humans of birth, maturity, off spring bearing, old age and death. For birds and fish and some insects, there are yearly migratory cycles. And for some animals there is the cycle of feeding and fasting; for animals and humans there are the body cycles of heartbeat, breathing, and organ function. There are civilization cycles, reincarnation cycles, and evolutionary cycles. Humans are currently moving past the sub-human state into higher consciousness and beginning a new cycle of much healthier and longer life spans.

The Universal Law of Love

The law of love says that love is literally the glue that holds the universe together. This glue or vibration continually surges throughout the created worlds, continually filling and flooding all of existence with this glue – this vibration – that comes from the Infinite Creator of the All, and it is done out of love for its creation. In a very real sense, it is this love vibration that keeps the all of existence going, and it is love, the emotion of self-love that keeps the body healthy and in hemostatic balance. All of the negative emotions of anger, rage, jealousy, and especially resentment (from stress, demands and pressure) create illness. Kindness is a facet of love, as is gratitude and especially compassion. To fully express self-love means that you will take care of your body's physical needs: exercise, dental care, quality food and drink. Self-love is providing for yourself financially, socially, and in partnering. Love means sharing your gift with others, being of service, and helping to make the world a better place. Love means to appreciate the gift of life and all of creation, to find joy in the life forms of the earth, and to look forward to all of the new discoveries that await you in your lifetime.

The Universal Law of Help

The law of help says when help is asked for it must be given. This is the reason that prayers work. The Creator designed Its creation such that for all of the lessor beings, if any being is needing help for anything, then that help must be given. Where does the help come from? We all have spirit guides and when you ask for help, your spirit guides reach out through interdimensional networks and connect you with those who can help you. And so, all problems can be solved. And this means that all health issues can be healed. Even aging can be slowed down, or even reversed. But the biggest mistake that humans make is that they don't ask for help. You must first ask for help before it can be given. So, with the Law of Help, there is no question that can't be answered, no problem that can't be solved, no situation that can't be improved. But you must first ask for help in order for it to happen.

The Universal Law of Karma

The law of karma says that all past actions are forever attached to the soul and any action of harm to another will create a karmic debt that must be repaid in the current life in progress or in a future life by receiving the same harm that was meted out, or by suffering from some affliction or illness. It is true that the Master from Galilee took some of the karma of the human race upon himself when he died on the cross. Karma is actually a gift from the Creator to give fallen souls a chance and a way to redeem themselves. Virtually every man and woman on the planet carries some karma. Karmic payback can manifest in some interesting ways. Today's police were often law breakers in past incarnations; today's medical healers were often warriors in past lives, and this is due to a requirement that souls have the opposite expression or opposite experience to balance out the overall soul life experiences. Karma has four layers. The first layer is the familiar, "what you put out is what you get back." The second layer is the karmic energy residual from past karma, i.e., the red nose of a teetotaler who was an alcoholic in a past life, or the chronic neck pain in one who had been beheaded in a prior incarnation. Layer three is the karmic obligation of the one who harmed another to be brough before his victim to try to redress the harm and damage he caused. Layer four is the karmic requirement that the evolved souls help the stragglers to prevent them from dragging down the whole human life stream.

The Universal Law of Opposite Expression

Opposite expression comes about because when higher dimensional light, energy, and consciousness comes down into our 3D world, it has to go through a prism and it separates into a spectrum of expression in which humans tend to see only the polar opposites instead of the spectrum of possibilities. Humans tend to categorize all things as polar opposites: good-bad, right-wrong, 'our way is good' – 'your way is bad.' Opposite expression is the reason that you can never get 100 percent agreement on anything, there will always be some who will take the opposite point of view. It is also a major source of world conflict in religious beliefs, in political issues, among corporate executives, among national leaders, etc. Opposite expression appears in human gender, male-female, in human achievement, high-low. The evolving human will choose to see and seek a middle ground position in everything such that the issue is for the good of all.

Survival Clocks and Humans vs. Enlightened Clocks and Humans

Most people are living in a deeply ingrained fear of moving beyond the confines of the box of spiritual dogma and political protocols. But we will challenge that right now and ask, "Is it possible that my life can be changed so that my life span can be extended if I could know about the new path of life extension?" Let us look at a historical timeline of timepieces. First, there were crude devices to measure time such as the sundial and water clock, then later there were hand wound spring watches and the fine pendulum grandfather clocks with all of those gears that you could see move. Let us for a moment go into a grandfather clock and watch how all of those gears work. It is amazing to watch how precisely all of the gears mesh and work together. The creators of these timepieces spent much time crafting every single gear and piece of them and all of the parts work together flawlessly. Uncannily, it's almost as if the pieces are evolved and enlightened and aware of the other pieces around them. It's almost as if they were alive as you see the windings and the clicks that happen in perfect synchronicity. One part moves to allow another to interface. It's so precise and beautiful. And the creators of them clearly loved them and made a plan for them to work in perfect precision that way.

But now, let us look at another type of watch or clock that doesn't work so well. The grandfather clock could be called an evolved or enlightened timepiece. Everything in it works in fine enlightened precision. But the second clock is a survival clock, which, of course, is a symbol (where one thing stands for another) or a metaphor for the current human condition now on the planet. It is emotionally hard to watch this clock (or unevolved human) because each piece does its best, but the pieces are not shaped quite right. Each piece doesn't seem to know itself or that it is part of a bigger plan – the clock. And in like manner, each unevolved human body part doesn't seem to know that it is related to and part of all of the other human body parts. But the clock still works and it survives, and the unenlightened human still survives, but not as long as it could if it were more enlightened. It's interesting to watch the pieces work together. Each piece is not aware of each of the other pieces and they bump into each other quite often. Now, you might ask, "How does a clock part bump into another part? Aren't they mechanically meshed together?" The gears of the survival clock are not quite the right shape and they break easily because of it. Instead of interfacing with the other parts of the clock with perfect precision, they will bump and grind, and eventually break. Some parts may actually be destroyed. Others will take their place and then go through the same thing. These clocks exist and seem to work, but they do so poorly, and it's stressful to keep them working, and they do not last as long as the first group of precision clocks do. And exactly the same thing is true for those humans who are in the sub-human category.

When the survival clock's parts don't know who they are or what they're doing, they simply survive as best as they can. They keep on ticking and working – poorly perhaps, but they survive. To go beyond the survival clock, or to go beyond the sub-human state, you first have to want to, and then you have to give yourself permission to do it. You'll need to look at many things such as: Did I have a past life? Did I interface with others (in a past life) who are also here now, and what does that mean? Can I use my intuition to find a better path that is clearer for me? Can I enhance my intuition to better know how to follow it? Can I control the idea of chance? Do I expect synchronicity? Can I evolve I evolve into higher consciousness? Can I create benevolence for myself every day? Can I control my lifespan? Can I live longer? All of these things are part of the enlightened human. The enlightened human knows that their life is blessed because it knows that it is magnificent in the eyes of the creator.

Most timepieces have evolved far beyond the mechanical gear types into the age of the digital electronic watches and they are incorporated into laptop chips and smart phone chips and these are much more accurate and their circuitry is an evolutionary leap above the old mechanical types, and that is also where the evolved human is headed. There are many levels of higher consciousness as Sri Aurobindo pointed out and we as a human race are headed for ever higher levels of consciousness to eventually become telepathic and be able to replicate new cells from stem cells. But the first step is to cultivate compassion.

Some Esoteric Things About Your Biology and DNA

Let us talk about some esoteric things about your biology and your DNA. Well, your DNA is going to start changing but your science won't be able to measure it because the part that's changing will be the 90% of your DNA that your science used to think did nothing (or was junk DNA). But that 90% is actually the manual of your gene production. Your DNA which is currently at less than 30%-35% efficiency will slowly begin to increase in efficiency. And a human whose DNA efficiency is at 88% is a master and a number of these have walked the face of the earth. And they could do miracles. But they were only fully functioning humans, and they always said, "What I can do, you can [learn to] do also." But it takes evolving into a master like they were. They were simply what we would call masters of the past showing you what can happen if you want it to. Your DNA will start to work at a more efficient level and your biology will start to cooperate more fully.

You will live longer, a lot longer, perhaps as much as three times longer. Your body will start to eliminate diseases that it could not eliminate before. Your primal energy field will build a bridge to your intellect. This primal energy field is more aware of your body's corporeal issues then you are and it's smarter than anything you have now. It represents DNA at its best, working to give you a full conceptual view of your own cellular structure and it is a self-diagnostic tool that is intuitive and accurate. Biology is going to change. Life expectancy will become much longer. But unfortunately, there are some who would say, "I don't want to live that long. My goodness, I know what it feels like at 70. Why would anyone want to live 300?"

This a very three-dimensional way of looking at it. A more evolved way of looking at it would be, "How would you like it if you could feel and look like you were 35 all the way up to 300?" That is what is at hand. That is what is coming. Your body will begin to rejuvenate itself far better than it does now when your DNA increases in efficiency. Can you conceive of this? It is important to know that the efficiency of your DNA is now increasing from today's 30% to 35% of being connected to your body's primal energy field template. It is increasing to 38% and even more as you move into greater and greater compassion and this allows healing to proceed better and faster.

Suggestions for the Life Extension Student

The life extension student should do the compassion meditation several times.

The life extension student should release their resistance to developing higher consciousness.

The life extension student should work on becoming liberated from powerful kleshas.

The life extension student should work with the 12 universal laws on a continuing basis.

Perfection Means On-Going Evolvement to Ever Higher Levels of Consciousness

CHAPTER 6
Life Extension Thoughts and Emotions

Oh, life extension lies mainly in the power of your mind.
But if your thoughts are mostly of the status quo kind,
Then (unless you change them) you will indeed find—
They create lives of struggle, peppered with disease,
And create the short lives that mankind lives and sees,
And if you don't evolve—you will age—oh please!

But if you can evolve above the sub-human state
You will have greater health and here I reiterate
That you will live longer and can extend your life
In this I will not hesitate to reaffirm and restate.

If you think you have to age, then you will age.
But if you think you can live longer, you can
And you can reset the gauge of your lifespan
And age not as much—oh yes—engage in this

And say, "Be gone my sub-human state, stay in the past
And do not cling," and really it is not such a hard task
To bring in higher consciousness—all you need do is ask

For compassion to flood your personality thereby rearranging
Your consciousness above sub-human into patterns engaging
A mental focus on 'we-ness,' oh yes, that is what is changing.

Also change your habituated thought patterns of short life lies,
And mass shootings and wars and threats that the media tries
To paint as the only real reality—but know that this is changing.
The truth is that the old way dies hard, but eventually it dies.

The new way—is to sing the life extender's song
But to do this, you must do the work of living long.
Make it playful—emulate the immortal masters of old
And in deed and word and song embrace life extension
Knowing all along that it is where you want to belong.

We all live with an aging program that resides in our mentality linked to our culture that creates an expectation to age in a certain fashion the way everyone else does, and this aging program creates premature aging. Your thoughts are fundamentally a product of your belief system—what you believe about something— and what you think you deserve, and what you think is possible, and what your expectations are. In order to support life extension, your beliefs about how long a human can live will need to expand. What you expect to happen is what tends to happens. Your belief system also is based upon what you think is possible or not possible. If you think life extension, or living to your potential natural lifespan of 140–150 years is impossible, then it is. I have already noted that Wikipedia has articles that list at least 100 people who are over 110 years old! Your thoughts follow your beliefs and so you will need to expand your beliefs about what you think is possible or not possible regarding human life spans. In addition, your thoughts also are coupled with what you think you deserve. You will need to create the idea that you certainly do deserve to live that long. And then fundamentally to really create life extension (to actualize it, or actually do it) you will need to create the expectation of it—the expectancy of it. This involves coming to expect it with a certain cockiness. You come to the point where you just know it's going to happen. Then it becomes a knowingness or knowledge. You just know you are going to do it, because you have learned how to do it, and that is all there is to it!

You know you will do it because you will have done many of the processes in this book. And because you will have incorporated some of the suggestions you will read about. And because you know that your body is designed to live more than 300 years. And because you know that you are fed false information, you are fed daily disinformation, about how long a human can live. You will create a foundational, fundamental expectation that you just know you are going to do it. And then you will need to plan on it. And as time goes by you will simply need to just let it happen because it will. Again, a very good tool to help you expand your beliefs is to use fanaticism and become quietly, internally fanatical about it. Internally, mentally, and quietly, create and maintain a determined, unshakable; yes, almost fanatical mindset about it that you are a life extender, and that you are going to extend your life and that is all there is to it, period! And then you will do it!

Now, I want to seed you to fire your willpower. A very good way to do this is with an affirmation. For at least a month, say the affirmation below every morning as soon as you get out of bed. But really, at this stage of humanity's development affirmations should be said every single day without exception. Every single day.

"I am becoming a life extender. I am learning the processes and the practices of a life extender. It is my dominant intention to extend my life. I am open to learn and use all that I read about and hear about to help me live a much longer, more productive, more fulfilling life."

Remember, the Universal Law of Thought is one of the twelve universal laws. The Universal Law of Thought says, "Thought is the creative force of the universe." And when your unswerving, dominant thoughts everyday say that you are going to become a life extender, you will!

Fire You Will to Become a Life Extender

Oh, what is it that starts the manifestation of anything?
It is your will to do – it is your willpower – it is this I sing.
Your willpower is the alpha and the omega of what you bring
Into manifestation—if your will is weak—you get but the sting
Of wanting it, but not getting it—and so, you should ring
Like a brazen bell, your will to do it, avoiding complacency.
Let life extension boldly be your chosen path for all to see.
Where lifespans can be very, very long and go on and on
And if your will is very strong, you can live long and go on
To become a life extension king or queen and just let it be.

Indeed, you are reading a book that contains much information and wisdom on how to extend your life—how to live much longer than you thought you were going to live— and how to live long enough to actually reach your human potential of 140–150 years. But, if you are only just curious about it, with a, "Well that sounds interesting, but...", then you probably won't do it. It will take a powerful will on your part to commit to doing it. You will need to commit to doing the work. You will need to do the affirmations daily. You should learn and work with healing diets. You should learn and work with the breath-work processes. You should learn and work with fasting. It would be good if you can master some of the fasting techniques. It is imperative that you start to do the affirmations. You should do all of the meditations and visualizations and energy exercises. You should work on all of these things in order to become a life extender.

But, even if you don't intend to reach your potential natural life span of 140 to 150 years, there is still much information to help you live a healthier and longer life than you thought you were going to live. If, at the present time, you think you only want to live say 100 to110, then there is still much you can learn in this book to help you do that. And for all those who are destined to reach their natural human life span potential of 140 to 150 years, it is imperative that they fire their will to do it. I have heard it said that if your conviction is strong enough about achieving any goal, then whether 99% of the population believes it is possible or not does not matter as long as your own conviction about it is resolute and strong enough. Indeed, even if 99% of the population thinks it is impossible, you can still do it, if your conviction to do it is strong enough! It doesn't matter what they think. If your will to do it is strong enough, and if your willpower to stick to it is dedicated enough, then you can do it no matter what any others may think about it. And for those who are really excited about the idea of true physical immortality and feel that it is very important for them to be able to stretch the boundaries out about how long a man or a woman can live into the immortality range of 300 to 500 or more years, the secrets of the immortal masters are presented in the last chapter of this book.

You will need to do the practices you learn about in this book for a certain length of time. One year was specified for mastering fasting by Babaji. I would say to plan on doing them for at least three months for each affirmation and meditation and energy exercise. You have to do them long enough so that they cognate and become a new program and a new way of life for you so that they can rewire the neurons in your brain into those of a life extender, and then it becomes who you are. And when you meld into the techniques and they become yours, it becomes what you do. And to restate it, it eventually just becomes who you are. Do them for at least three months. Even consider doing them longer! Do them until it becomes your on-going way of life. Do them until it becomes you. When you reach this plateau, you can see yourself as a different person then the masses. You can differentiate yourself. You can see yourself as a master. You can say, "Well, I am a life extender! The others are merely mass consensus reality statistics." And then you will literally be different. You will have differentiated yourself from the others.

The most important first step in becoming a life extender is to create your willpower to do it. And your will-power to want to do something follows your excitement about it. You tend to do what you are excited about. Does it excite you to live and stay in good health and high vitality for 140 to 150 years? Does it excite you to eventually become a grand, youthful looking mature longevity master who can live 140 to 150 years? Does it excite you to become a way-shower for the rest of the human race to become the new human who will extend his or her life to live past that 150-year marker to live over 200 years?

Most people think that if they make it to a ripe old age that they will be a weak and wobbly, crinkled and crumpled, cranky and grumpy humanity who barely has half of their body functions working anymore. But you will learn how to become a youthful older person who lives in high vitality, high acumen, with every body function working just fine. I want to add that your later years can be your best years. Most people have more financial security in their later years. And you will have gained much wisdom from your past mistakes and choose to not repeat those again. And because of this you will be better primed to enjoy your later years. Why deprived yourself of your later years by leaving early, and by this, I mean passing away before you reach 115 to 125 as an absolute minimum.

You should begin to distance yourself away from the media now. The media: TV, newspapers, magazines, movies, etc. will all parrot the status quo life expectancy beliefs and media addicted people will age in concert to those beliefs. And media addicts are also the sickest people on the planet because they buy into the bombardment of scary ads that wave disease flags around to get people to spend money on some supposed remedy.

It should be noted that the more advanced information about the power of thought talks about thought in a very systematic way. There are major problems with negative thoughts because they create negative thought-forms, and these thought-forms want to (and tend to) impulse their creator (the human who created them) to act out the subject matter of the thoughts involved in their creation. So, there is much to learn about the power of thought and why choosing only positive thoughts is imperative.

The Laws of Consciousness and Aging

Now let us talk about the concept of consciousness and ask what is it? It is expected that the next stage of human evolution involves expanded and enlightened consciousness. But what is consciousness? Consciousness in not matter, it is not a physical thing. Unlike light, which has a speed limit of 186,000 mile per second, conscious thought has no speed barrier whatever. We must state here that consciousness represents a great paradox to scientist and philosophers because they cannot express it or describe it in any physical form. It should be stated that consciousness has many similarities to the Creator mind and the energies of the Creator. As close as it is possible to define consciousness, we can say that it is on the subatomic level, and that it is an energy field, a field, a force field of energy. And as such it can be transmitted. And one of your lessons and missions in this lifetime is to work with the relationship of consciousness to physical matter.

Can consciousness affect physical matter?

Indeed, it can and that was one of the major discoveries of quantum physics. In their experiments with sub-atomic particles, scientists could see that if they expected a particle to go up it would, or if they expected it to go down, it would. This is a crucial demonstration because it clearly proves beyond a shadow of a doubt that your conscious thoughts can and do affect physical matter, and this is especially important when it comes to your physical body and life extension.

If you consciously think that your body will live longer, it will. If you consciously think that you can youth, you can. Part of the laws of consciousness says that it is linked to your subconscious mind and to your unconscious mind. Therefore, your conscious thoughts are sent to your subconscious and your subconscious receives all conscious thoughts as instruction. Your subconscious attempts to manifest and parrot what your conscious thoughts are. That is why affirmations are so important. Rhyming affirmations are very good, because your subconscious mind loves a rhyme (that is why rhyming songs you like stay with you so long).

It is important to understand that to reach the higher dimensions and higher consciousness, you must begin to purify those thoughts of yours that will be sent to your subconsciousness so that they are of higher thinking. Consciousness can transcend the space-time continuum. That means it can transcend space and go beyond time. And you do this all the time in your dream states. Consciousness can also transcend aging. And that is the beauty of programming your conscious thoughts to – 'stop the aging program' – directly into your subconscious mind. And using affirmations to seed your subconscious mind with life extension instructions works because your subconscious mind affects your consciousness mind which, in turn affects matter, and your body is matter.

Extended Life Spans Are on the Way

After humans had crossed the Armageddon marker of 2012 safely, the spotlight for human evolvement began to shine on humanity for increasing human longevity. And predictions are that humans will now start to have better health and longevity mostly because they will reach a better balance in their emotional life and in their thought processes and in their physical bodies. So, attaining a better balance in your emotional life and in your thought processes and in your physical body, and in what you think is possible are the keys to extended life spans.

Your Body Is Designed to Live Over 200 Years

Life extension will begin to happen partly because humans will begin to realize that their bodies are designed to live much, much longer than they do now. You will begin to hear this from so many different sources that humans are designed to live over 200 years and actually even much longer than that to well over 300 years. And humans will finally begin to believe it, and then accept it, and then actually begin to live it. It is very important for you to know that short life spans basically come from false programming and low fear consciousness. As a man or a woman now on the earth you are constantly exposed to false media and societal and parental programming throughout your life. At birth you identify with your parents and their expectation of what is possible or not possible. They apply these beliefs to themselves and to you and you buy into it. You buy into their resentments and their tendencies to expect rule by force, rule by others and even violence, and almost all of rules that you grew up with are not altruistic and for the good of the whole. They are almost always without exception for the good of those who are in power and for who have the wealth. And most important, this issue of humans wanting power over others to point of using force through armed conflict and battles and eventually war is one of the main causes of short human life spans! This is all low consciousness. This is all sub-human consciousness. And one of the real problems of low, fear-based, sub-human consciousness is that it has kept the human DNA working at only about 30 percent of what is possible. That is why humans age as fast as they do. This low consciousness that all of mankind is operating at now is not anywhere near its potential.

False programming in your news media will give you an idea of how long humans are supposed to live without any notion of the divine driving force that exists in every human that has the potential to allow humans to live 3-4 times longer than they do now. And because you are fed this fake information over and over and over again about aging, and because everybody else believes it, you buy into it too. There are a few places in your media that are beginning to tell you the truth, by saying that you can give instructions to your body about how you want it to perform. You can give instructions to your body to slow down the aging program. But, one of the major reasons for the short life spans of the current time frame now (10 years past the 2012 Armageddon marker) is in your belief system which says you can only live so long, and it is an actual fact that it is your belief system that ends your life!

You and all of humanity are living this story which tells you that your maximum life span is only about 90 to 100 years! That story will be changing and it is already slowly starting to change now, but for all to believe it, it must change within the mass consensus reality consciousness. You will understand that it will have to do with living in a state of harmony most of the time. It will have to do with the nurturing momentum that is taking place now of ensuring that everyone will be taken care of no matter what their skills and abilities and handicaps are. This will start to happen within the next generation or two, and it will increase in the generations after that. This will all take some time—and estimates are that it will take 200 years after 2012, or it will take until about 2222 to finish the human longevity upgrade. We know that seems like a very long time, way beyond your life expectancy, but those of you who really want to can stay here that long.

You can start it now. You can start by imagining and creating an expectation that you are going to live at least 110 to 120 years. It is much easier on your belief system to go for an intermediate age like 110 or 120 instead of 200 when you start this. And then as new things to help people live longer begin to come out and make their appearance, you can increase your life span goal and add more years – 130, 140, 150. And when real rejuvenation starts to happen and become available, wow – what then! Perhaps 200 years, maybe 300 years, 400 years? Also, the immortality secrets of the masters as revealed later will show you the practices of the ancient masters of physical immortality that will also let you live that long. And in one hundred to two hundred years from now the new rejuvenation technologies may make incredible lifespans available for the first time since Atlantis.

People Are Programmed to Age

Indeed, it is important to hear that there were many times when humans lived at least 300 of your years, and if you look at your physical body, it is designed for that. So, let us ask again, why do you age? Some of it comes from your belief system which is the actual energy you feed your brain that tells your body that you will only live this long. Although that seems very simplistic (and it is much deeper than you understand at this time) changing your belief system is the key. Average life spans were once in the 300-year range, and there were even times when humans could even reach 900 years! It is vital to know that your health and aging are a product of what your society tells you, and this is blatantly regarding the influence of your media. Advertisements in the media clearly tell you that if you are a certain age then here's what's wrong with you, and you need to get this or that expensive treatment so that others can profit. When messages such as this are watched over and over and over again, they go right into your subconscious and become a new program of beliefs. When this happens, your life extension is thrown right out the window. But this is what your whole society believes and this is a powerful reason why people age like they do. But you can begin to stop all of that. And the first step is to wean yourself off of watching TV! This programming is not only on TV, but it is also in other forms of your media including your newspapers, magazine articles, and especially ads, and it includes your movies, and it is even seen in many your performing arts that have a negative story line ending with early death. Why are there no story lines ending in happy, healthy, very long life spans? Now, you are going to need to reverse all of this, and you can begin to reverse it now. Here is an affirmation meditation to get you started in reversing it. In all of these affirmations, speak them out loud but in a low voice. It needs to be spoken loud enough for you to hear it. Speaking it out loud to yourself works with the Universal Law of Speech, which says, "speech will be used to influence." You should go to a place where you won't be disturbed, you should move into your meditation posture and slow your breathing; you should visualize your body, its cells and your primal energy field permeating them, and it would be a good idea to bring in your spirit guide team (your own spirit guides, the angles and ascended masters).

Affirmation Meditation for Health and Life Extension

"I am a powerful and I know that I can create new programs and beliefs systems that my body will follow. My body and all of my cells and my primal energy field, I am speaking to you now.

Cells, body, and primal energy field, I want you to hear this! I remind you that your normal and natural state is health and to be balanced. There is no need for disease of any kind. There is no need to age like the masses do either. Cells, body and primal energy field, I want you to stop this premature aging. It is totally unnecessary. I am telling you now that I want you to go on a new program of regeneration and to go for my natural life span potential which is at least 140 to 150 years!"

Your Body Can Live Over 200 Years

Again, we need to remind you and reiterate and make it quite clear that your body is designed to let you live far beyond 200 years, and yet human don't make it anywhere close to that. Men and women don't live long enough yet – they don't even come close to 200 years which is a fraction of how long your body is designed to let you live. Humans don't currently live long enough to remember any of the profundity of the changes that have taken place in the past 200 years. Your grandfathers and grandmothers would be very impressed with the freedoms you have now that were impossible to them and were not allowed to them in their day. Our human lifespans today are ridiculously short. Did you get that – ridiculously short! We only live a fraction of what we were designed for. We just don't live long enough yet. If we could live 200 years (a fraction of what our we are designed for) we would be able to see the patterns emerge. We would start to be aware of the potentials and not just expect a repeat of the same dysfunction of the old conflicts and the wars. We would be able to see the start of human evolution into higher consciousness. We just don't live long enough yet. If we could live 200 years (a fraction of what our DNA is designed for) we would begin to see the patterns of humans evolving, of humans rising to higher levels of consciousness. And then we would then become aware of the potentials to rise to a higher consciousness as a whole planetary civilization where war is not an option anymore – where war becomes a non-option! And then we would not just expect to repeat the same old dysfunction and destruction of war. Then we would all want to live longer. And then we would all start to live longer.

You Will Need a Meaningful Purpose for your Life

Now to reach your current natural lifespan potential of 140 to 150 you will need to have some purpose for living that long. You will need to have something meaningful to do with all that extra time. You will need to lay out what you want to achieve in those 140 to 150 years. I would like to see you start thinking about that right now. This gets you smack into your ideas about retirement. Why would you retire at a certain age only to travel and idle along? And you will need to think about supporting yourself for a much longer life span than conventional retirement planning. What is the purpose of only traveling and idling along? Are you supposed to stop doing everything and go have fun for the rest of your life? This is following conventional programming and this will kill you. And many of you already know this.

It is fine and even perfect to shift from doing what you were doing and then start doing something else of a needed and creative and worthwhile nature, but to stop and do nothing but play the rest of your life will end your sojourn on the planet very quickly because it means you are finished. Once everything is completed, you go. You leave. There is no judgment about it and there is nothing wrong about it but it simply means that you have finished your work. So, when you plan to stay on to reach that 140-to-150-year life span potential, you will need to do some serious planning about what work you want to get done with that amazing amount of extra time. And that is all there is to it.

The biggest reason for human life extension will have to do with humans in mass reaching a higher consciousness where everyone knows that the whole of humanity is the simply sum of each and every one of us, and so for each and every one of us to be happy and taken care of is a high priority item. When you start to rise to a higher consciousness level by beginning to see benevolence in all that is about you (instead of fearing that you might be harmed by something about you), then you can give your body instructions for a longer life.

When you cross that threshold of going from lower density and transition into higher consciousness, then you can even begin to rejuvenate yourself! You may wonder why you need to rejuvenate your physical body because you will eventually be leaving it anyway – but the short answer is that you have the opportunity to claim mastery in this. You have the opportunity to master many things and one of the most important of these is your physical body. You may start getting ideas about how you can work with not only the earth and everything about the earth, but also about your own dense physical body as well. The earth and you are related. When you start getting these ideas, you can even eventually rejuvenate your body. And remember, that eventually you will start to get the notion that this idea of perfection means mind over body mastery and when you evolve enough you will get the idea that indeed, you can rejuvenate yourself just by the purification of your body and the purification of your mind and the purification of your emotions and by intending that you are going to rejuvenate your physical body.

Your Media Gives You False Beliefs Daily

We are as a human population beginning to evolve into a newer higher consciousness where eventually we will create peace on earth and we will be functioning better than ever before. This is not to say that there are not, of course, many unevolved, dark areas in our world. There are and they will continue for a few more generations. But let us look at where we are as a world society and most important where you are in the scenario of fake news today? What have you been told you cannot do? What does modern medicine say is going to happen to your society and you at your age? This is all dis-information. Your medical science instruments cannot measure the magnificence of your consciousness or its healing power. How long are you supposed to live? Disinformation in your news media will give you a ridiculous number, something like 80-100 based on a body without any divine driving force. Your slanted news will tell you that you are supposed to "drug up" because you're over a certain age. This is all nonsense news. We have said this before. When your media gives you these kinds of things, turn it off or stop reading it, or better yet get rid of your TV and become media free to avoid all the fake and nonsense news that is bombarded at you every day. And begin to get into your liberated potential. I tell you this––your natural life span is 140-150 years. I tell you this––your body is actually designed to live much, much longer than that. Really, it is designed to live far longer than 300 years and it has a design template of 900 years. So, it is important to start believing this and break away from the daily false short life media bombardment.

Without Your Bias, Your Body Design Is to Let you Live Over 900 Years

But we don't. So where does your body take its cue from? The answer is—it takes it from the past. Isn't it time to change all of that? Basically, you can actually live far longer just by telling your cells that all is okay and by not buying into the negative things that you are told by others. The chemistry in your body responds to both positive and negative instructions. Give your body instructions that the future is always a good one and that good health is expected and that you are re-framing the past and eliminating the fear of all disease. This will help your body to overcome the bias it has that the future will somehow be bad. It is very important to overcome this bias. I dare you to visualize yourself in your place of perfect peace and do the following meditation! Assume your meditative posture, command your body to stillness, and regulate your breathing to a slow metronome type of rhythm. Bring in your spirit guide team. Project yourself into your place of perfect peace and feel that there is no time, no space, no form – just you and your consciousness being there. Then speak in a low voice to your past bias. This is an important affirmation-meditation. Read it several times to partially memorize what you are going to say.

Meditation to Reprogram Your Bias

"I am in the unknown. My past bias, get in the back seat. I am driving now. My past bias, get in the room of old things where I can shut the door for good. Only new positive things are allowed now. I don't know what they are but I program them to be good things and benevolent. My body, my biology, my past, get in the back seat and stop giving me old, fearful information or old ideas about short life spans and about a bad future. It's time for the great escape from all of that. It's time for me to have and expect a great leap in life span and a very good future where only good things are allowed to happen. It's time for me to plan on life extension to a good life of at least 140 to 150 years minimum! I can finally get to that place where I can say, "You know, it's so good to be alive." I'm stepping into a place where I haven't been before and no matter what people tell me, I finally trust my intuition, and I'm finally out of fear, and I finally know that I can live to be at least 140 to 150 years old now without my old biases."

Let's Talk About Life Extension Now

What happens when all of your cells start to change now because they are presented with a harmonious energy of thought? What happens when there's a confluence of energy that aligns things for the first time? What happens when one can assume a perfect stillness that represents an absence of emotional-mental conflicts? What happens when one can concentrate the mind on allowing the life journey to go on and on and ever on? What happens when you can think about allowing a continuation of your life instead of an ending as you do now? What happens if you are 60 to 70 now and start to have life extension thoughts that say, "Well, I am only at one half of my life cycle, because I expect to live at least 140 to 150 years, so I have 70 to 80 more years left!" And this doesn't factor in rejuvenation which will be coming in a decade or two.

All of these are the things that create health, long life, happiness and balance. It's the discovery that inside you is a force to be reckoned with that comes equipped with a DNA package from the original creation. A fast track to the great escape from short life spans is to see a God who loves you, through every situation, and who will take your hand if you allow it and protect you, and keep you safe in all situations. This is the best escape of all because it helps you to balance all the other layers and layers of bias and filters and history of the past that you will have to get through to escape the old expectations of the short, disease-ridden lives of your past.

Can you instruct your body like that? Here is a rhyming mantra that may help you to seep it deeply into your memory banks. You should say these rhyming lines several times

Good bye to my old past life bias of short lives and fears.
Hello to my new beliefs saying I can live 140 to 150 years.

As the Masters knew, these three: (body, mind, emotions) are the key to immortality.

You should know that the design of the human life span template is to live over 900 years!

CHAPTER 7

Bad Memories, Sexuality, and the Future Human,

The spotlight for human evolvement has begun to shine on increasing human longevity. This will take some time. It may take until 2212 for human longevity to reach 200 years, and that seems like a long time in the future, way beyond your life expectancy, but those of you who really want to can stay here that long. In the last chapter you will learn the secrets of the ancient immortal masters who did live 500 to 900 years. And you will learn how it is possible for you also to develop the mastery that they had and do the same thing. As we have said again and again, one of the major players in this idea of human longevity is your belief system which says that you can only live so long, and in actual fact, it is your belief system that ends your life! Indeed, you and the rest of humanity are living this story which says that your maximum life span is only about 90–100 years. That story will be changing and it is already slowly changing.

Getting Rid of Bad Past Life Memories and Welcoming Good Past Life Memories

Higher consciousness will prevail over everything and it is possible to rewrite (and higher consciousness is about rewriting) the memories a human remembers from a thousand past lives. Yes, you can do this! We are going to take those past life beliefs and traumas and nightmares—from the ways that you died, and the children that you've lost, and the wars and battles that you've fought, and all those that you've killed, and all those who've killed you—all of those bad past life memories that seem to resurface and rescript your expectation of what your future holds into fearful imagined scenarios of destruction, limitation and a sense of hopelessness. Your past lives were typically short, fearful, and contain uncountable awful memories of horrible plagues and wars and tortures and intrigues and killings. Clearing these past life traumatic memories is very, very powerful and is even what some of those who are highly evolved do using their own methods.

And also, amazingly, clearing those past life traumatic memories can even clear some of your own health issues and allow you to youth! This past life soul-memory postures everything that is you including the way you think, your personality, the way your body accepts a disease, how you view your self-worth and even your spirituality. When you do the exercise below, you are about to turn the corner on how your body sees the earth today. Read this meditation several times so that you can recall the basic theme of it for both the bad memories and the good memories. Then pick a time and a place when you won't be disturbed, go into your meditative state, perhaps bring in your spirit guide team, and become perfectly still and speak in a low voice the theme below.

Clearing Bad Past Life Memories and Celebrating Good Past Life Memories

"My past life soul memory, my cells, and my brain, all of which are me in this incarnation and also me in a thousand past lives – now listen to this! There is a change, a big change, and I am directing the change! I am in command! I am in charge! I need all of you to pay attention to what I command!

I command that all of the bad things – the negative memories from my past lives stop coming up – the horror and the betrayals because they are no longer serve. I command you to cease and desist those thoughts, ideas, images, beliefs and emotions that are beneath me as a spark of the Creator God. I command you to stop playing the old tapes of betrayal, sorrow, bad feelings, and anger that I've experienced. I am in charge of this and I command this – I command it to stop!"

"But I also command that all of the good things – the beauty, the joy, and the wisdom that has happened to me in a thousand of my past lives with the maturity of my soul surface in ways that will surprise me with benevolence in good things and positive expectations! I command you to see the beauty and benevolence and God inside of every cell of my body. Let my past-life-soul-memory record only show the best things that ever happened to me, because I am in charge and I have spoken!"

Oh, the old negative past life memories are still there, but they will stay there, and this gets you past the problem that almost everyone on the planet has and that is that you think you are not in charge of your life. But, in fact, you do have complete control of everything in your life including your past life memories.

Sexuality and Life Extension

Oh, it is your birthright to delight in the dance of the night.
The height of ecstasy is to relish the dance of the night.
The closest one can come to the Infinite Creator of the All
Is in the orgasmic experience for the human race – the small
So that humans can savor the moments of the clouds and the rain
Which is the ecstasy of creation and do it over and over again.

Sexuality, is one of life's greatest pleasures. Indeed, not only is the power of the sexual drive the only reason that you and I are here, but it is a constant and continual force that is always looking for creative expression. Sexuality equals creation. Sexuality equals continual life expression. Expressing your sexuality on a regular basis helps you to extend your life. There are several reasons for this. One is that is it strongly negates the death urge. Who wants to end their life when they are enjoying sexual pleasure? Most people when they are enjoying their sexuality would think, "Wow, what if this could go on forever!" There is almost no desire to die prematurely when one is having great sex. And so, the death urge gets banished when couples enjoy their sexuality. Another reason is that sexuality stimulates a greater secretion of hormones that foster body maintenance and assist longevity. This is why older people who express their sexuality often have less gray hair than those who don't. You can almost tell those who are expressing their sexuality and those who are not by how old they look. A third reason comes into play for those who have achieved an enhanced ability to fully allow and experience their total range of sexual sensations. When one is able to cultivate this skill, to let their full range of sexual sensations blossom then another facet is added that carries over into life extension. A special gland if it is stimulated enough through enhanced lovemaking will secrete even more substances that can greatly improve the skin, complexion, and other parts of the body to create something of a rejuvenation affect. Most people don't allow their full range of sexual sensations to blossom. But it is possible and it allows for a rejuvenation potential.

Many young people don't get as much as they could out of their lovemaking because they don't talk about their sex life with their partner. Most couples could get more out of it if they would communicate to their partner and tell them what they like, what pleasures them the most, and what they would like their partner to do differently. Communicating with your partner about your sex life together is important in being able to enjoy sexuality to its fullest.

Many older people who have lost a partner feel left out of mainstream social life with its emphasis on the younger set. They often feel alienated and somewhat outcast and the idea of expressing their sexuality may seem like a distant possibility at best. If a partner has been lost, they should grieve over it and then let it go. "Oubliade, oubliada, life goes on…," as the song goes is a correct statement of life and the sexual drive goes on as well. There are many examples of older people who have gotten over an earlier relationship or two and moved on to a new one to continue their sexuality and companionship. Of course, one needs to attract a partner. And to help with this, fitness and flexibility and looking good are helpful. This is another reason why regular fitness and yoga workouts are a good idea.

Expressing your sexuality on a regular basis is very healing. I was given a dream in which a kind but firm voice said words to the affect that if a person can allow themselves to be loved more (and let their sexuality express itself more) then their own health problems will not be as severe. The sexuality and the life extension connection are very clear. Although there have been immortality schools where sexuality was absent, (and it can be done) most would agree that the more satisfying way of reaching an extended life span is with a partner that you can share your sexual pleasure with. The sexual stimulation will also secrete hormones and substances for both you and your partner to help you both reach an extended life span.

Extended Life Spans in the Future Human's Day

In the future human's day, ten generations or 200 years beyond 2012, futurist or seers (those who can receive visions of the future) say that the future human will have an entirely different belief system and a completely different way of relating to others in his or her culture, and the future human will have a far greater knowledge of the higher aspects of his or her body then humans do now. And hear this, because of all of these things, the future human will be far more careful about the thought patterns he or she allows and the emotional states that he or she creates. When we learn more about how the future humans live, we can begin to start being like them and emulate them.

Predictions are that humans will start to have better health and longevity mostly because they will reach a greater balance in their emotional life and in their thought processes and in their physical bodies. Partly it will be because humans will begin to realize that their bodies are designed to live much longer than they do now. People will hear this from so many different sources that humans are designed to live way beyond 200 years that they will eventually begin to believe it and then accept it and then live it. They will understand that it will have to do with living in a state of harmony most of the time. It will have to do with the nurturing momentum that is taking place now of ensuring that everyone will be taken care of no matter what their skills and abilities and handicaps are. This will start to happen within the next generation, and it will increase in the generations after that. And the biggest reason for human life extension will have to do with humans in mass reaching a higher consciousness level where everyone knows that the whole of humanity is the simply sum of each and every one of us, and so for each and every one of us to be happy and taken care of is a high priority item. And that will create a joy for life and a zest for living that missing in our time now all over the world.

Today's human cannot define the master number of 44 or the higher master numbers after that (55, 66, etc.). These have to with evolved thought where you more consciously choose the kinds of thoughts that you allow and you more consciously choose the more enlightened and spiritual thoughts. These higher master numbers will have to do with choosing to stay in the emotional state of contentment most of the time. They will also have to do with increased wisdom where you know that forceful conflict never resolves or solves anything. These things all have to do with common sense, maturity and wisdom. But more than that, a sort of knowing will start to happen and it will be accepted as the new way of things, and it will be called the new human nature and the new human. This will be reflected in what the public wants to have in their movies and on television and on the internet.

Slowly, but surely, the old energy will be eliminated just like grade school was eliminated. And along with all of this, the propensity for health and long life will blossom, and much will be revealed and changed to allow that to happen. The knowledge that all things recycle and the appropriateness of lessons learned will give you greater wisdom. The future human's spiritual development and maturation is based on service. Life itself is a gracious act of service. Or stated another way, your life is not only about you. Many of you have strong resistance to making this sort of a shift in consciousness. To get from the dark side (of war) to the enlightened side (of peace) there are profound transitions that need to happen. What you will have in the future is a planet where humans think very, very different than you do today.

A Day in the Life of a Human in the Year 2212

Let us follow a day in the life of a future human who lives approximately in the year 2212. This is ten generations past 2012. Futurist paint a picture of an entirely different reality that people will be living in then they do now. By the year 2212, the futurist sees that people will have literally changed their relationship to everything around them – to God, to people, to everyone else around them, and to the earth. In the future human's world, ten generations beyond 2012 in the year 2212, benevolence will have become the king of the emotions. Futurists see a world where vast changes will have taken place. They see a world where everyone is taken care of. They see a world in which peace and happiness have become the human experience, expectation and norm. They see a world where humans have made a great leap in life extension and many are already living 200 years. They see a world of future humans (in the year 2212) who were born into a world that has long stopped thinking that all help comes from the outside. People in their day do not believe that they are unworthy in the sight of God. Absent is the idea that they must call upon a higher source or authority to solve or accomplish everyday life problems. So already we have a huge difference from the way most people would see things now.

Futurists predict that by the year 2212 most of humanity will have come to accept that all things spiritual and beautiful are carried inside of them. "God is inside," always has been the message from the masters, and by 200 years in the future it will have become an accepted fact and it will be applied in everyone's everyday life. Therefore, the rush to find help from the outside that you see today will be totally gone. The deeply seated notion that humans are somehow always unworthy and that all good thing come from above will be long past. It is predicted that by the year 2212 the Biblical saying, "made in the image of God," will come to be understood as, "made in the image of love." And in the future human's day humanity will realize that "made in the image of God the Creator," or "made in the image of love," has always been inside. Therefore, humans can access God, spirit, and the ancestors instantly through built-in processes. So, with this background we will start the story of a day in the life of a future human who lives in the year 2212.

He wakes as always and gets ready to go to work. He puts both feet on the floor and the first thing he does every morning – **<u>every single morning</u>** – is to say his daily affirmations to expect good things to happen. This is the very first thing he does every day! He pushes the consciousness of benevolence through his day right at the very start. His affirmation to expect a good day might go something like this:

"This is going to be a good day for me. I am going to have a consciousness that will surpass any challenge I may have today. Any challenges I have will have a most benevolent outcome for me. Good things are always before me."

Today many humans would say, "Oh this is going to be another one of those difficult and maybe horrible days. I hope I survive it." Can you see the big difference in this? The biggest difference is that the future human has a built-in expectation of benevolence, but there is even more. The future human is really saying. "I can control this day to be a good day in which everything that happens is benevolent and I expect that everything that happens will be for my best good!" This is very practical and it is the very first thing he does when his feet hit the floor. He celebrates the fact that he can get through any problems that may come up. What he is really doing is creating his reality for that day! He is creating through his consciousness something physical – a bubble you might call it – that goes with him—that goes before him wherever he goes. He is creating a benevolence bubble! It is actually as practical as dressing for work. Is it too much to think that you might start doing this too? There are people today who are starting to do this. They use the term MBO, for Most Benevolent Outcome. They start their day by creating an MBO bubble for themselves just like the future human. You can start to do this too. Indeed, you can.

Next, the future human dresses, brushes his teeth, and leaves in his vehicle for work. He works for a worldwide telecom corporation in an industrial park. And just as he arrives at work, he sees a woman who is sobbing and is staring at one of the large overhead news screens that are common in his day. He overhears what happened through the audio system. The screen shows an air vehicle crash with the flight number. The woman knows that her two children and her husband were in that air vehicle that crashed and killed everyone aboard. The magnitude and impact of this tragedy was so powerful that when our future human saw it, it even had the potential to change his life forever if he lets it. A horrible event has just occurred– he sees a crying woman, a mother and wife, and there are others around her who are trying to calm her and comfort her. In the background he sees the large overhead screen that shows the crash and those who are carrying away all of the dead and covered bodies. Life for this woman has just taken a terrible turn. There is the potential for her to have life-long grief. Her day started out well, but in an instant her children and her husband are gone—and there is the potential that she will carry this day to her grave. Now, our future human takes all of this in and he is overcome with sadness and grief and he starts to weep. Yes, he weeps with compassion. You see in his day, in this new world of 2212, in a very practical way, compassion has become the king of all emotions.

Our future human takes in all of this in and suddenly there is more than just empathy that comes from him. His sense of compassion (and telepathy) is so well developed that he can actually feel everything she feels. He leaves the scene and goes to his office and continues to weep quietly at his desk. And then he does something that is very special. He gets hold of himself and then starts a process that he knows very well and has done many times before. He begins to visualize this woman in her future as she is recovering, understanding and surviving and eventually having some peace over this event in ways that are not understandable today in our current psychological understanding. He visualizes this woman recovering in so great a manner that he visualizes her laughing again. This is the visualization that he sends her directly to where she is at that moment of her horror and grief, knowing that he has just practiced what will be called, 'compassionate action.'

If this happened today, there are those who are also very compassionate, but their compassion might actually get the best of them and wound them forever. They would never forget the sight, and it would affect their inner child and would dampen their own joy factor and this very likely would cause them to age! Indeed, in today's civilization, there are so many things that happen every day that are like that, there are so many horrors and tragedies that happen every day that many sensitive humans empathize to such a degree that it ruins their own lives. All they can think about is how unjust things are and how they want to change them. And this pulls them down to the lower energy of worry and fear. And they will die younger because of it! They have let their compassion get the best of them.

But our future human does not let that happen. No, he knows better. He knows that is the bad way and also very dangerous. So, what the future human does (that is not dangerous) is to see a situation like this and then go into compassionate action. The future human never left his desk. But he immediately thought of a solution and sent actions of compassion because he knows that consciousness can change things. It is like today when you might pray for a person. But it is much more than that. He projects joy in the future for her. He creates understanding and recovery for that woman, letting it begin that day. Can you begin to see yourself going into compassionate action in your own way, but not getting directly involved? The future human stops weeping and starts smiling because he can actually see it happening in his mind. There will come a day when she will laugh again – not today, or tomorrow, or next month, or even next year. But there will come a time when all these things will be settled in her in her own way. He participates in the humanness of her recovery even though she remains by the overhead news screen.

Our future human is soon having a nice day at work, but a half an hour later, he hears the cheering. One of his friends in another cubicle in his office had just gotten promoted to one of the positions that he wanted. Our future human wandered over to be part of the celebration and he fully participates in it, and he meant it. He was pleased that his friend was succeeding and he was so pleased that that his friend got a promotion and raise – he was so pleased! He didn't see it as a reflection of anything to do with himself. He didn't let the news affect his happiness for his friend at all. This is almost inconceivable in our time now. In the old energy of our day, there is way too much self and ego projection. "Why not me? What did he or she have that I do not have? He took my job. I am not going to talk to him anymore. I am going to go home and sulk for a whole week, maybe a month, maybe a year." Some at this point would do anything to stay depressed. Our future human might have thought, "This is awful! I find out that somebody else got the job I wanted and got promoted instead of me." But this was not at all the reaction of our future human, because, you see, he had a very strong belief that "benevolence and good things always happen," and because of this he was able to feel joy for his friend. His telepathic abilities were so well developed that he could actually feel the joy and happiness emanating from his coworker, and he was so happy for her. Here in front of him was a friend who had something wonderful happen, something that was good and would change the person's lifestyle. He knew that his friend would soon tell her family, and she would have a beautiful dinner and sing celebration songs. Our future human thought what a good time this is to celebrate the joy of his friend! Is this even possible today? Can humans really put away feelings of hurt to the degree that their first thought is to celebrate the one next to them who got the job they themselves wanted? This, my friends, is the evolution of consciousness that is coming! You see, just like our future human felt empathy for the woman who lost her children and husband, he also actually felt the joy (telepathically) of his friend who got the promotion. It had become so built into him over generations of evolution.

It will seem today far beyond what a human could normally do, but it's coming in the future.

The next thing that happens is that his boss is on the video phone and asks him to come into the office. His boss gives him some bad news that will affect his future at work. Now as our future human leaves his boss's office, just for a moment he is flooded with the old energy of worry and fear. What would he do without his job? How would he tell his wife? What does it mean to him? Then the future human becomes still and takes a deep breath, and in an instant he re-frames everything that happened and realizes that it is the beginning of shift or a change. And more than that he knows beyond a shadow of a doubt – **he knows beyond a shadow of a doubt** – that it will be a good change for him, a benevolent change, because he programmed it that way at the very start of his day. He programs it that way at the very start of his day every day. During his early morning affirmations, he created the energy of benevolence that surrounds him at all times. He doesn't know the timing of any of it, but he actually starts to smile because he knows that it is the beginning of a shift, a change, that is going to be good for him. If this happened today, what would be the typical reaction? It would be this: worry, worry the whole next day, worry the whole night, worry the entire month. Tell all your friends so they can worry with you. This is drama. Whatever happens, happens but the drama continues. It would build a bridge of darkness between employer and employee. They do not appreciate me, they do not want me, etc., etc. None of those things were on his mind, but he had to convert all of that potential in about three seconds from an old-energy fear reaction, to a thought that is way above the consciousness level of today. He automatically shifted the energy into a scenario that said, "Maybe I do not belong here. Maybe this is a sign. Maybe something is going to happen that is beautiful. I can hardly wait. I will do as I am told. I will work overtime. I will even accept the pink slip because I know that there is something better coming!" Can you the reader begin to think like this? It is quite a culture shock, isn't it?

"He could have thought this is awful! First, I find out that somebody else got the job I wanted and got promoted instead of me, and then I get the idea that I may not be employed anymore." But this was not at all the reaction of our future human, because, you see, he already knew that "this or that something else better was coming," because he had a very strong belief that "benevolence is always coming, and that good things are always coming, and that good things are always are always before me." Our future human already knew that "this or that something else better was coming," because he had a very strong belief in benevolence. His thought processes always ran along the line that "benevolence is coming, good things are coming, and that good things are always before me." He did not know when or how or any of the timing of it and the timing was not that important. The important thing was that he knew **beyond a shadow of a doubt** that whatever was going to happen was going to be good for him.

Now our future human is going home. And like all humans everywhere he had a lot on his mind but a distant thought said that he had forgotten something, and when he arrived home, he knew what it was – it was his anniversary and he had forgotten to get his wife flowers. This brought up a dilemma. His wife would get upset if he wasn't home at the usual time for dinner, but she would also get upset if he didn't bring her flowers to celebrate their anniversary. Immediately he had to make a decision. Should he make a run to the flower shop, get the flowers and a card, and come back, late for dinner? Which was better? Being late for dinner, or not having the flowers? Our future human's intuition gave him the answer right away to go, not to a distant flower shop, but to a nearby flower stall, and so he went there, bought the flowers and the card, and went home, albeit fifteen minutes late for dinner. He did not know what would happen, but he had the flowers and the card. Now, he could say, "Happy Anniversary, honey, I'm sorry I'm a little late for dinner," and so that's what he did. But something else happened. His relatives were there. His wife had organized a surprise anniversary and a birthday party to celebrate their anniversary and the birthday of one of their relatives. He had the flowers in his hand. He was not late for dinner because there was no dinner. There was a party instead and they were all going out to a restaurant. He had not disappointed his wife, and he had the flowers. What happened was that our future human paused to listen to his intuition, a higher part of him that knew beyond what he knew what was going on at his house. Today, some might call this a future-self bleed through, or Deja vu, but in the future, it will be called using your intuition in a heightened way. His intuition knew what he should do and he listened to it and he trusted it. He immediately went and got the flowers. In our time, in our unenlightened world, a human might have a 50-50 chance of making the right choice, not understanding that there is a higher part of them (a future-self, part of them) that knows the best choice. There is a higher self above you and for our future human, and this higher-self part of him knew that there was a party at his house. Listening to his intuition was common sense for him. He used it every single day as a staple, not something that fleeted by without substance. It told him who to call and how to say the things he had to say to others that he needed to talk to. It was his way of life and he knew it worked. He had practiced it for a lifetime and he trusted that it worked.

After the party was over, his wife said, "Thank you so much for the beautiful flowers. We had a great time!" Our future human agreed, and the furthest thing from his mind was to tell her what happened at work. He smiled and thought, "I'll give her the good news later." He was about to go sleep. His feet were on the floor and before he lifted them in bed he said, "Thank you Creator. Thank you for letting me be there for that woman. Thank you for letting me help my friend celebrate. Thank all the cells of my body for youthing today. Thank you for the disease that was chased away today because I did not go into worry or fear or drama. Thank you, inner child and intuition that I can smile now. I am not worried about my job because I know that this or that something better is coming." He looked at his life partner and said, "Good night sweetheart, thank you for being in my life."

This story is real. This is the way of higher consciousness. This is the way of the evolved, enlightened human. This is your potential future and you can start the momentum towards becoming a future human right now. Even though it seems unreal or impossible, these things in the future human's day define enlightenment. This is coming. The age of compassion is coming. The age of enlightenment is coming. And it will re-write and re-frame everything that humans think about, react to, and do. And it will also include great life extension. This is a snapshot and it is in your future lineage. This is your potential future and if you will work on it, you can begin to create a benevolent life for yourself right now and a life that also has great potential for life extension. It would be very good for all of you to re-read this chapter several times and do the exercises below to bring you a bit closer and closer to the future human state. They will start you on the path of becoming a future human right now and they will open the door to a greater life extension potential.

Exercise 1, Creating Daily Benevolence

What is the first thing the future human does upon getting out of bed? He or she says an affirmation that creates a benevolent outcome for all of the situations he or she may face during that day. To begin this path, say an affirmation like the one below in a low voice the very first thing in the morning – **every morning** – as soon as your feet hit the floor. *"Today will be a good day for me. I am going to have the consciousness that will overcome any challenges I may face today such that the outcome is good for me. Good things are always before me and only good things will come my way, because I program it that way. I request an MBO (Most Benevolent Outcome) bubble to surround me at all times for any issues I may face."*

Exercise 2, Giving Compassionate Action

Begin to incorporate compassionate action for those who cross your path who are in obvious suffering. Be very careful to not get directly involved with them for that will lower your own energy. Instead, send them a visualization something like the one below directly to them where they are at the moment of their suffering knowing that you have just practiced what will be called 'compassionate action' and at some point, in the future it has the potential to help them. *Visualize an image of them in which their suffering is gone, or has become alleviated, or visualize them as being happy again and thought project this vision to them. Visualize them being happier and good things happening to them and thought project this visualization to them.*

Exercise 3, Letting Go of Self-Centered Ego Reactions

Begin to command your ego to take a back seat and allow yourself to actually feel joyful at the success of others when before you would have felt resentful of their success. Learn to actually begin to feel (telepathically) their happiness. In your own life when someone gets something that you might have also wanted, speak in a low voice, *"I command that my ego and selfish self-interest yield to allow me to be able to feel the joy and happiness of others and to participate in their happiness when good things happen to them."*

Exercise 4, Redefining Bad News

Begin to redefine what you would label today as bad news into simply there is a change coming and I know it will be a change that is good for me. It will be a change for the better because I have programmed it that way. When a situation in your own life happens that you would have labeled bad before, say in a low voice, *"This is only a change that is coming and I know it will a change for the better because I have programmed it that way by creating an MBO benevolence bubble that surrounds me at all times."*

Exercise 5, Developing your Intuition

Begin to develop your own intuition by sensing what would be the better choice in situations where there may be several choices. Say something like, *"Intuition, would it be better for me to take the time to drive to the store to get something I need, or would it be better and save time to look for it at home?"*

The Importance of Increasing Your DNA Efficiency Level

We will seed you with this idea in this chapter and give you some basics about the importance of your DNA efficiency level, and in the next chapter we will give you greater depth on it and a meditation to begin to start it. We have said this before but you may need to hear it again – human DNA is literally quite amazing. It is what connects you to your soul and to the consciousness of the earth or Gaia through your primal energy field which in turn connects the DNA of every one of your trillions of cells to each other. Most of humanity's current DNA efficiency level is quite low, only at about 30% due to the old energy of fighting, machismo, and intolerance – and the old energy on this planet is filled with thousands of years of war, a very long history of war. That is the main reason why human DNA efficiency is so low. When you are born, at the moment of your first breath, the quantum part of your primal energy field looks at the earth's crystalline grid and adjusts its DNA efficiency to match that of the planet. And that is a large reason why your DNA efficiency is so low, only 30%. When your distant ancestors were on the planet in small numbers they were in touch with Gaia, and Gaia responded and so did their DNA which took its cue from Gaia on how well it worked or at what efficiency level it worked at. The earth and humanity work together. The earth and humanity are linked together.

And in the last 40 years humans have been working closer to Gaia and this is now being registered in the new children and that is why they already have the higher DNA efficiency of 35%. The DNA blueprint of humans is designed to work with Gaia and Gaia is designed to be reactive to humans. They form a Human-Gaia system and one will always affect the other. The energy of the earth is ready to send the signal to the old souls who start to understand all of this so that you, as an old soul, can take charge and begin to change your own DNA efficiency and your own primal energy field through the templates that float in them – hear this again, you can start to increase your own DNA efficiency level and your own primal energy field through the templates that float in them.

You can do this on your own by raising your own consciousness level by creating compassion for Gaia, and for all of the animals, plants, humans, for yourself, and for all life. And after that by stating with your pure intent that it is a dominant intention of yours to raise your own DNA efficiency level. You can change the quantum print or efficiency level of your DNA with compassion and with your pure dominant intention to do so. And as we have said your DNA is designed to give humans a very long life and it is designed for full rejuvenation and self-healing. Your DNA is designed so that the bridge between you and your primal energy field is always there. There are accounts in your scriptures of humans of old who lived very long and very healthy lives. Did they really? The answer is yes because they knew that their primal energy field around them and the others of their day was so aligned with Gaia that they cooperated with and shifted with Gaia. It is what the ancients knew and it is one of the main reasons why they were one with the planet and were able to live so long.

This is something that humanity will start to do also in our own current times. One of things that you can do to start this process now is to observe the children. Notice that they are coming in with different conceptual attributes and they don't think in the same linear fashion (that this event must always follow that event) that adults do. This will be noticed more and more and will become the new norm, but we can also change our thinking patterns and habits to be less linear and more spontaneous and to even encompass things from the interdimensional realm. And as time goes on there will be a more efficient DNA that is able to create the missing link between your primal energy field and your normal human brain. And when this happens it means that you will have more intuitive thoughts coming from your primal energy field about what will assist you to live a longer and better and healthier life style.

Some of you will have an impulse to change your eating habits as if you are tuned into your own cellular structure that seems to say to you, "You know if you substitute these new foods for what you usually eat and drink, you're going to live longer." The result will be instinctive eating changes that you will not be able to explain. Also, habits that you've had for years will start to drop away because your cellular structure will help you start to eliminate them because it knows that they no longer serve you and will shorten your life. If one of those habits was overeating it may surprise you to learn that your cellular structure may make metabolic adjustments that bring your body into line. Other habits that your primal energy field and more efficient DNA will help you drop are addictions to substances and when this happens it is an allowance that will indeed let you live much, much longer. You will also begin to see changes in the cellular regeneration of your body that will surprise you. You will begin to heal faster and you will know it. You will notice that you are starting to get sick less often even though the prevailing belief is that older people are supposed to get sick more, but you won't and then you'll notice that something is changing in you.

So, all of this is saying that you can also begin to have some of the same attributes that the new youngsters have. And you will also slowly awaken to the new energy that is on the earth which will allow you live longer. Your DNA will start cooperating in a more efficient way and increase to perhaps 35%, and for some of the old souls perhaps even to 40%! And your DNA can even be on its way to something much, much higher. Master Jesus, Elijah, and Buddha had DNA working at least 88%. There are emotions and energies within humans that are catalysts for enlightenment and one of the main ones is compassion. Indeed, it is compassion, for when you truly have compassion, your heart opens wide and you are filled with emotion to the point of weeping, yes weeping and having tears in your eyes. That is compassion and it is thick, very thick with emotion.

And you can also claim your own healing because you are starting to get in touch with and connect to your primal energy field. When you hear about those impossible healings from spiritual organizations what happens is that DNA goes 100% for only a moment. But that is enough to cleanse the body of the disease. So, why don't you do that right now? If you can imagine it, you can have it. See and create an image of yourself with pure cellular health. It serves Earth dear human for you to live longer than you think you're going to live. But you might want to know how can you begin to do this. We will give you a meditation in the next chapter to help you begin to increase your DNA efficiency.

Also, it is important to realize that raising your DNA efficiency level is directly connected to attaining a greater enlightenment quotient so to speak. You should practice the future human exercises and have a good idea of what attaining a greater enlightenment would mean for you. Work on developing the future human traits. What would it be like for you to be able to send compassionate action to others in their time of need? What would it be like for you to be able to have an ever-present, overpowering feeling that only good things are allowed to happen to you throughout your day? Could it be possible for you to be able to feel joy at another person success when you also wanted the same thing? Are you able to use your intuition to always choose the best path when there are several paths to take?

Also, before doing the meditation to increase your DNA efficiency, google DNA and the cell it is in and memorize what they look like. And when you do your DNA efficiency meditation it should be done outdoors, and you should work on and strive to sense a connection with Gaia. Also, it would be good to ask your spirit team: your spirit guides, the ascended master and angles for help when doing the meditation.

CHAPTER 8
DNA Efficiency and the Death Hormone

Oh DNA – it is a most important major body part.
Its design, extremely complex is a real work of art.
The human genome has three billion base pairs
Of DNA's twisted ladders with many steps and stairs.
Inside almost every cell it holds instruction sets
That code for replication – the complication gets
Immense – a multitude of long chain proteins
Are made from millions of DNA micro machines.
But all of this is in the 3D view that humans get.
DNA has a much more magnanimous role even yet
For DNA is interdimensional and has layers twelve
And each plays a special part that mankind can delve
Into and fully fathom for they have been revealed,
And in them are your soul and your primal energy field,
And your body blueprint, but the last two as wisdom tells,
Aren't linked well enough to replace old cells with stem cells,
But when higher consciousness is reached this will come.
And a new immortality will arrive when all of this is done.

Coherent DNA = Higher DNA Efficiency = Life Extension

What happens to a human group when they have nothing in common with another human group? They tend to separate and even war with each other. What happens to humans who find that they all have the same thing in common? They tend to unite, share resources, and celebrate what they have. Do you see how this can affect the human population on earth? If the study of all things and how they worked revealed God inside of everything, wouldn't that tend to unite everything? The common denominator for all things is love.

DNA is very special. It combines all sciences. It has multidimensional attributes. It is quantum and at the atomic level. It is locked with all of the other DNA in your body, and it has seeds of the creative Source within it. It has the memory of all that you ever were, and all that you will be in it. But at present it is not coherent. However, eventually it will be. Now this begs the question, "What is coherent DNA?" Coherence means that something will vibrate in tune to a driving vibration and this is seen when one tuning fork causes another one to vibrate at the same frequency. Multidimensional DNA, if it has coherence with certain specific dimensional attributes will create literally magic. This is because this coherence will start to seemingly evolve. And it is important to note that the difference in evolved DNA can extend your lifespan four-fold — yes indeed, four-fold! The difference between DNA working at 30 percent efficiency and DNA working at 90 percent is a dimensional alignment that will eventually be called coherent DNA. This is all a part of the evolving future human.

Some of the attributes of the evolving future human are that there will be ways of hearing and seeing and reading that you cannot even begin to imagine today. You will begin to discover that God, the creative Source, is in everything. Consciousness and love are the glue of life existence. Several factors that can apply to consciousness can affect change. Did you know that as the physics of consciousness is explored and the wisdom factor is applied or gained by 'passing the wisdom barrier,' that what happens next is an exponential understanding and application of the rules of consciousness that creates a factor that generates benevolent action? When you reach a point of understanding the physics of consciousness – how it works, the mechanics of it, the distribution of it, and the spiral delivery of it – then you shut the door on older energy. It's an almost exponential evolution. You will come to be born wise. You are now at the wisdom barrier and have just broken through. The benevolent factor and the wisdom barrier all work within the laws of the consciousness of physics in ways that you will indeed figure out that will end up creating an increased DNA percentage activation and this will increase generation after generation after generation. Eventually you will have a human being who can manipulate matter and seemingly create something out of nothing! It's just physics. Doesn't it make sense that a multidimensional physics can control a lower dimensional physics. And creating something out of what appears to be nothing can be done eventually by humans in a highly concentrated meditative state. And it can also be done through the application of the inert gas technologies.

Peace on earth. What will happen when a civilization without war can create anything it wants and no one ever goes hungry? What would it be like to live three or four times longer than you do now and have good health through all of it? What would it be like if humans could put themselves into a quantum state and ascend briefly into higher dimensions and go anywhere in the world they wanted? This exists.

Coherent DNA = 4 Life Spans

It's the attitude of benevolence in creation – intelligent design and more. God is in the atom. God is in all matter. God is in everything. God is why everything exists. This understanding will slowly lead to a new human coherence with each other. Also, human consciousness is an attribute of multidimensional physics. Human consciousness – that elusive energy – will be seen as multidimensional quantum physics that has laws and rules of its own. Laws and rules that can be understood, applied and used. And all of this will have to do with working with and learning to feel compassion and benevolence and love to a much greater degree, and feeling one with Gaia and wanting to heal her, and feeling love for all other humans and wanting them all to be healed and happy. It will have to do with feeling love for the animals, the plants, the planets, the stars and yourself. It will have to do with evolving into a higher coherence where you are able to achieve a higher calmness and stillness then you ever could before, and this reflects an ability to free yourself from emotional and mental conflicts. It will have to do with evolving spiritually and maturing in wisdom. We, as a human population had evolved enough that by 2012 we were able to bypass the 2012 Armageddon marker and not unleash the Armageddon back then. And now as we move forward in time when we become able to create coherent DNA our life spans can increase 4-fold!

I had a glimpse about what that might mean – what coherence with the creative Source might really mean during a morning exercise in the park when after tossing peanuts to the squirrels, I understood that it meant that I was able to feel love for the squirrels as I watched them, even as I saw them each trying to hoard the peanuts that I tossed them and keep the others away. I found that I could still have love for them even though they were not evolved enough to able to share for that was simply the way they are. They are not evolved enough to share. It is also the way most humans are too. But I could still feel love for them and for all of the creatures in the park. And then I reflected on the saying that we humans are made in the image of God, and the real understanding of this is that it really means that the image of God is the attribute of love, for God created the universe out of love. And we humans were created with the ability to have and feel love. And this love creates a coherence with the creative Source and this coherence with the creative Source creates a coherent heartbeat for me and for all other humans who can come to understand this and work with it. We can feel love for all in creation even though we can see that many are unevolved and have imperfections and some even have negative intentions.

The Ancient Masters DNA Efficiency Was At 88%

Some of the ancient immortal masters of old as they evolved have attained a DNA efficiency of over 88% percent and when that happens, they became almost immortal, because at that level of DNA efficiency their stem cells were activated and their stem cells created new cells for a new rejuvenated body bypassing what happens now where your existing cells replicate but each replication is less and less accurate and causes aging. So, as these ancient masters matured and evolved spiritually, their DNA efficiency began to increase – to 44%, 54%-55%, 66%, 77% and 88%. When humans reach 88%, they actually start to meld with their soul. Where is your soul? It is in one of the interdimensional layers of your DNA. It is in every chemical in your body. It resides in the energy of your consciousness in ways that you don't know. It is accessible in ways you don't know and it loves you beyond measure. If you could think of the most beautiful color, you've ever seen that would be the wrapping it comes in. If you could think of the most benevolent force, you've ever felt that would be the door to your soul. If you could think of the most love, you've ever had from anyone, it would be the opening words it would speak to you. It surpasses anything you have ever experienced on earth.

When you reach 88% you become almost immortal. You are designed to be divine. You are designed to live almost forever. Your design is renewable biology. Every cell keeps going and going, especially with the divinity within you. When your DNA starts becoming more and more efficient, cellular rejuvenation creates new cells from stem cell blueprints, not copies as it does now. This 88% efficiency DNA cellular structure never really gets old. When you are at 88% you never get old! And that is where humans are headed. But all of this will take some time. Futurist see it just beginning to happen in about 10 generations (or in about 200 more years).

Recap = 88% Efficient DNA = Radical Life Extension

Mankind on the Earth is a young race. We have passed the threshold of 2012 when we as a planetary population decided that we were not going to unleash the Armageddon. However, we have a long way to go before we reach full maturity. When we have finely and firmly reached full maturity such that it is a guaranteed given that we will most assuredly not self-destruct through our horrible nuclear weapons —when that happens, we will have attained a DNA efficiency of over 88% percent. And when that degree of DNA efficiency is attained, you become almost immortal, because again at that level of DNA efficiency your stem cells – yes, your very own stem cells – become fully activated and they create new cells for a new rejuvenated body and this totally bypasses what happens now where your existing cells replicate but each replication is less and less accurate and causes aging.

When you begin to create coherence with the creative Source, you create coherent DNA which as we have said before will extend your life four-fold. Hear this again – coherence with the creative Source will extend your life four-fold! Basically, when you create the attribute of benevolence in your daily life experience – in your own daily life experience – you will bring in intelligent design into your life and that is benevolence. You will come to know that God is in each and every one of your atoms. You will know that God is all matter. This understanding will slowly lead you to becoming the new human, the future human who has a coherence with each other and one another just like future humans, and begining to work on becoming like the future human is a first steps to helping you to increase your own DNA efficiency level.

When you hear it several times it may begin to resonate with you that human consciousness is an attribute of multidimensional physics and as such can work with multidimensional quantum physics that has laws and rules of its own that can be understood, applied and used to create matter out seemingly nothing (actually out of the aether) by attaining states of complete stillness, intense concentration on a thought-form, and pure intent. Yes, you will eventually be able to create any form of matter you want out of the aether just like master Jesus could do. You will also come to know that your DNA is very special. It is a combination of all sciences on the earth. It is multidimensional, it is quantum, and it has God within it, and it also locks into its memory all of your past lives, all of your present life, and all of your future lives! It is the most complex multidimensional creation that exists on earth. And you will eventually come to understand and know and create coherent DNA. Multidimensional DNA, when it is coherent with multidimensional benevolence will create a great increase in human life span. Benevolence is the key. When multidimensional DNA has coherence with and vibrates in resonance to states of equanimity and serenity and blissfulness, and when fear becomes something of the distant past, and when compassion for all of creation becomes your daily way of life, then your DNA has evolved. When human DNA evolves like this, it will literally extend life spans four-fold!

The difference between DNA working at 30% (which it is now) and DNA working at 88% is a dimensional alignment that can be called achieving coherent DNA. We will say it again, at 88% you will actually start to meld with your soul. And again, when you reach 88% you become almost immortal. You are designed to be divine. Because of the inherent human potential to create coherent DNA, your basic body blueprint design is to let you live seemingly almost forever. Your design is renewable biology. Every cell keeps on going and going and going, especially the divinity within you. When your DNA starts to become more and more efficient, your cellular rejuvenation will create new cells from stem cell blueprints, and not make copies of itself as it does now. This 88% efficient DNA cellular structure never really gets old. When you are at 88% you never get old!

And we repeat, all of this has to do with attaining higher consciousness. So, it is imperative that you start working with the practices that will lead you to higher consciousness: greater compassion, much more harmony, greater coherence of all of your body's systems, and the ability to create a much greater love for yourself and for all of creation, and expecting benevolence and only good things to happen to you in your daily life. Compassion and benevolence and love are really the keys. And when this starts to happen there is a great outpouring of new inventions and new ways of living that are so benevolent that today they can't really even be imagined. And that is yet another story all by itself to tell later, but it is another reason to hang around and extend your life. And all of this is where our future is headed.

Doing the future human exercises are basically prerequisites for doing the meditation below for raising your own DNA efficiency level. When you feel you have been able to incorporate the future human abilities to some degree you may be ready to try the meditation below to raise your own DNA efficiency level. You should practice working with the five attributes of a future human: (1) you strongly feel that benevolence is in your day and life every day, and you expect only good things to happen to you because in your daily affirmations you create it that way at the start of your day, (2) you ae able to send compassionate action to others who are suffering, (3) your ego is much less and you are able to feel joy in others success when before you have only felt resentment, (4) you are able to redefine 'bad-news' into only a change is happening and it will be a good change because your benevolence expectation is so well developed that you know that it has to be something good for you, (5) and you have developed your intuition enough so that it leads you to choose the best choice in situations where there are several choices.

Meditation to Raise Your DNA Efficiency Level

Become very calm, bring in your spirit guide team, command your body to stillness, and go into your meditative state. Feel that your own consciousness level has risen. Feel strongly that you expect only good things and benevolence to happen to you this day and every day because you create it that way through your daily affirmations. Feel that you have developed compassion for the people in your daily life – your partner, your coworkers, your local universe of fellow humans, all humans, all animals, plants, and all life. Feel your connection to all humans is benevolent. Feel your connection to Gaia is growing stronger and stronger. Feel that your ego driven "I-centered" behavior has begun to transition towards a "we-centered" behavior. Feel that your intuitive abilities have increased. Feel that your DNA is multidimensional and that it has coherence with and vibrates in resonance to states of equanimity and serenity and blissfulness. Intuit that fear is appearing less and less in your daily life. And intuit that compassion for all of creation is becoming your new daily way of life

Now create an image of just one cell on your mental screen. It can be of any tissue. Move to that cell's DNA. Now speak in a low voice to your primal energy field, and speak to this cell's DNA, and speak to your body as a "we-ness" team and tell them all that you want your DNA efficiency level to increase as much as your light quotient allows. Begin to intuit that it is it happening. Begin to create an expectation that it will happen. Stay in your meditation awhile. Then slowly come back knowing that your DNA efficiency will start to increase to a higher efficiency – to a greater linkup with the templates that float in your primal energy field. And begin to intuit that your DNA efficiency is increasing to a higher percentage level as much as your light quotient evolution will allow.

Now when you do this meditation, relate to what the words say. When you say you want your DNA efficiency level to increase, it means that you are going to start doing the things that will allow it to happen. It means that you will start to work with Gaia and do meditations with Gaia. It means that you will start to feel love and compassion for all of the animals that inhabit the earth with you, and perhaps feed the birds and the squirrels. It means you will start to work with compassionate action for those who have fallen or suffer without getting directly involved with them). It means you will drop your ego a bit and begin to want all others to find happiness. It means you will redefine bad news as only a change is happening and it has to be a good change for whatever it is because you programmed it that way. It means you will develop your intuition to a higher level so that you know what is the best choice for you to make when there are several choices to choose from.

Stopping the Death Hormone Release

Your DNA has an Instruction Set That Ages You

Did you ever wonder why all humans all over the world always start to age after they reach their maturity of about 35-40? Well, this has been revealed and here is the reason. There is a death hormone that starts to be released when humans reach their maturity at about age 35-40. Even medical science sees this in what they term the aging substances that old senescent cells release, but the full story is far more involved and complex than that. Before 2012, human DNA was only working at one third of its potential. But after 2012, the spiritual awakening of humanity is accelerating at a much faster rate, and you can apply the wisdom learned from all your prior past lives and what you've learned in your present life. There are some important details of your DNA that most of you are not aware of yet. Science does not yet see the magnetic instruction sets that are contained in your DNA. It is not mentioned in mainline literature and, of course, it is certainty absent from medical science, and yet it is one of the most important parts of your body. This magnetic imprint is upon the chemistry of your DNA, and this huge magnetic imprint is responsible for the way you look, the remembrance of how your body grows, and the seeds of your life itself, but this huge magnetic imprint also has... unfortunately, a very real instruction set for your own termination. Indeed, it does. It is there and it tampers with and greatly reduces your life span. It actually makes your life less than one-tenth as long as it could be without it!

Your Primal Energy Field

We have talked to you about your primal energy field before but now we will speak about it in greater depth and detail. All humans have a primal energy field that is extremely important concerning the aging and death cycle. It may be elusive, unseen and not even known by you or humanity or your science, but it is there and it is this field that connects all of your cells together to communicate as one unit. It is your backup system that keeps your heart beating even if the spinal cord has been severed. It is your backup system within the DNA field that keeps you alive. Even if the spinal cord is severed your DNA field is connected through your primal energy field to your brain, and then your brain's signals are communicated to your heart muscles and digestive system through your primal energy field. It is a body wide energy field system that knows more about your body than anything your brain knows. It knows about your nervous system more than you yourself could ever know. Your primal energy field is everywhere in your body: it's in your hair, it's in your toenail, it's in all of your DNA. But it has a real instruction set for your own termination.

You Can Stop the Death Hormone Release

These words are not spoken lightly. We tell you that you have great power because we will tell you next how you can change all of that. But first we feel that some background information is in order and should be given. It was decided a very, very long time ago in the higher realms by the overseers of planetary development that long lives did not serve the learning process of the humans on earth, and so the death hormone was implemented to allow for many short lives each followed by a reincarnation. Next, it is important to distinguish between your human brain, which is programmed for your physical body's survival, and your primal energy field which is programmed for your spiritual survival. Let us look at what spiritual survival means. In the old program (before 2012), in the Age of Pisces, spiritual survival meant giving humans many short lives which was the engine of enlightenment at the time. Your primal energy field by design will give you short lifetimes, because short lifetimes fostered spiritual growth back in the old energy before 2012. This death- rebirth cycle was the engine of enlightenment back then. And so, for many thousands upon thousands of years that has been the way of it – slow spiritual growth through the birth-death cycle. This is because in the older consciousness, the recycling of souls was key to the slow path of spiritual enlightenment. In other words, humans were given short lifetimes to have experience, and then recycle back into the planet (though the death-reincarnation cycle) so that the wisdom they learned could be used and applied in succeeding lifetimes.

Without the Death Hormone Release Very Long Lives Are Possible

But you should know that now, without this instruction set the human body can live a very, very long time—for over 900 years! Some ancient masters have demonstrated this. Yes, over 900 years! Today these magnetic imprint instructions cause the interruption of your natural rejuvenation cycle and the result is aging and death. In order for this death substance to be released, there has to be a clock, and indeed, yes there is a body clock. In the DNA and genes of every cell in your body there is a chronograph, a mechanism that counts, and unfortunately, it is this that creates your own termination. It is the catalyst for death. In your life cycle when you have reached maturity, unfortunately, the body clocks in your cells strikes the hour for the gradual release of the death chemical. The death hormone is released on schedule from the 'body clocks' in your cells and it is this death hormone that interrupts regeneration and rejuvenation and causes aging. But the death hormone was created for a time in the age of Pisces, and the age of Pisces has now come to an end and the new age of Aquarius is coming in.

And the system of short lives is changing and is also coming to an end. This system of long lives is coming in now in the new age of Aquarius, and there is a huge change afoot that says you don't have to reincarnate anymore. Instead, you can remain here as your DNA starts to increase in its efficiency and by the time it reaches 36% (in numerology 36 equal is 3+6=9, and 9 means completion of the old death-reincarnation cycle), you can stay here for a very, very long time.

You can stop the aging program in a very profound way. But to do that you will have to work at it. You will have to work with your primal energy field because it doesn't know that yet. Your primal energy field actually works to the old program which, as we have said, is the 'death and reincarnation cycle.' And the faster the learning curves are, the higher the potential is for humans and the planet to move into a higher vibration and make a leap to higher consciousness—and this equals and equates to spiritual evolution. And one of the main things to learn in the new energy after 2012 is the benevolence of everything and a profound compassion for the gift of life and the gift of creation and for all of creation.

Longer lifetimes are the key to the human and to the planet's evolution. The old death-rebirth cycle is inefficient in the new post 2012 energy meaning death-rebirth and having to go through the process of growing up all over again. Most of you can see that you could accomplish so much more on the planet if you could choose to stay here and live a double lifespan, or a triple lifespan, instead of age and die as you do now. Some of you will think that this is impossible but that is simply old traditional thinking. It is possible, and we will now give you a meditation-instruction-set on how you can avoid this mechanism of the 'body clock' and the 'death hormone release.' It is very important to say this instruction set out loud but in a low voice to activate the Universal Law of Speech. And it is also important to pick a time and a place where you won't be disturbed. And it would be very beneficial to bring in your spirit guide team and ask them to help you with this. It is going to take some wisdom and understanding on your part, and some compassion for you to change all of this in the new higher vibration energy in order to avoid the 'body clock' and the 'death hormone release,' to become able to stop the aging and death cycle.

You Will Need to Reprogram Your Primal Energy Field

Very important – and a major key to stopping aging is to reprogram your primal energy field! It is designed to age you, even though your cellular body is actually designed to rejuvenate you (which is on hold now until you reach a higher level of DNA efficiency). The fact is, you can reprogram almost everything and anything in your body. Many of you have already made changes to your personality, to your human nature, and even to your cellular body structure. Now we are going to work on: first your primal energy field; and then second, all of the cells in your body individually; and then third, your whole body as a 'we'-ness collective whole.

When you do this, it will be the job of your primal field to change all of that, and stop the death-rebirth cycle and initiate the life extension and rejuvenation cycle. This is very important and we will repeat it. You must talk to your primal field as though you were talking to your best friend. It will listen. It is reading these words with you right now. When you talk to your primal energy field and give it the credibility of intelligence to listen and understand, it will. That is the credibility you must have with it. And only you can do this. You must give it the signal to change. You need to learn how to communicate with it. Your primal energy field is your smart body and it is time for you to reprogram what it thinks is your spiritual survival. This is because it did not cross the 2012 marker like your consciousness did. Recalibration of your primal energy field is not automatic.

Now the beauty of all of this is that you don't have to convince your primal energy field of anything. It knows. It has been waiting for the call. As soon as it sees the progress you've made in raising your consciousness level, it is a done deal. Did you hear that? It knows who you are. Remember it is your smart body. But it doesn't know what you want until you make the call. The result of this is that you have the potential to live a lot longer. It is also very important to integrate and see all of your cells as being integrated, working together as a team, and vibrating together. Your cells will understand the new instruction set you are going to give them because they too are all involved in the body clock. Unless you, and all of your cells vibrate together, they will never know what to do with the death hormone. So, it's the 'we' that is central to eliminating the death hormone and to self-healing and to life extension and to rejuvenation. All of your body parts are part of the whole. Verbalize in the affirmation-meditation below the 'we-ness' of all of your biology. Honor your body and all of its parts and all of its cells as a 'we-ness' whole. Now, never verbalize or think doubts about this or about your seeming inability to do something. Do not speak doubt. Instead conjure up a certain cockiness that you know good and well that you can do this, and that the time is right for you to do it, and that your higher consciousness wants you to do it. Now, let us do the following affirmation meditation to stop the clock and death hormone release.

Verbalization is crucial to this entire process. It's due to the fact that your biology, your intellect, and your spiritual side have all come together to speak words as sound that all of your body's cells can resonate to, and can understand, and can begin to follow. We will say it again – it is that important. One of the twelve universal laws is the Law of Speech. This universal law says, "Speech will be used to influence. What you speak is what you influence to create." So, speak very firmly in a low voice and in a very plain and instructional way.

Meditation to Stop the 'Body Clock' and 'Death Hormone Release'

Go into your meditative state, slow your breathing, become very still, and bring in your spirit team and ask them to help. Speak out loud in a low voice and say to your primal energy field: "My primal energy field, please listen up because I am speaking to you. My primal energy field, I acknowledge you and your intelligence, and I want to befriend you. Dear primal energy field, by my intent, I choose to disconnect from your magnetic short life imprint. I want to tell you that I no longer have to die to create spiritual growth, because I am already on a rapid spiritual path. I want your old programming of a short life to drop away. I want a new program put in place that will allow me to stay here on the planet for a much, much longer life time—for at least a double lifetime and even more. I give myself permission to have this magnetic imprint deactivated now! It is no longer appropriate, it is no longer needed, and I cannot allow it to prevent me from doing what I came here to do and need to do."

"Now, I am speaking to all of my body's cells and I am instructing them that we as a team are going to halt the release of the death hormone and deactivate the body clock."

"Now, I am speaking to my whole body as a 'we-ness' whole. Dear body, in all appropriateness and sacredness I am addressing you. We are together in this lifetime, and together we will heal ourselves and we will choose to move forward into our new contract to live a long, long life and move into life extension. Together we will rejuvenate and together we will have power over the clock and over the death hormone release." Indeed, and so it shall be.

Dear reader, we as life extenders are now moving way past the old paradigm (before 2012) that says when you get up there in years that you will have health problems. It doesn't have to be that way. You can also program your primal energy field to keep you healthy as you don't age. And you can also youth, it is not that complicated to youth either. It is indeed possible and it is filled with love. This is new and it is also smart enough to work well. You are in control of so much more than you were ever taught. And when you start to do these reprograming exercises you are going to start to see it happen, and then you'll start to believe it, and then you'll start to live it. Your life is important and your longevity is important and many of you have work to do in healing the planet and helping to heal all of the humans who live upon her. It is crucial to humanity and planet to move into a world brotherhood and sisterhood where benevolence is king and unity is queen and where humans live much longer than they did in the past, in a new world harmony that the planet has never seen before.

Much new wisdom has been recently revealed to help humans live far longer. New revelations on life extension have dramatically increased. The masters of old were aware of the non-physical aspects of what in their day was called physical immortality, and in our day is called life extension in the 200 to 300, year range. The ancient masters called it perfection of body, thought, emotion and spirit. In our day the cultivation of compassion and benevolence becomes paramount. And so, when you can feel compassion for Gaia, for yourself, for your family members, for your coworkers, for all of the people on the planet, and for all of the animals, plants, stars, planets, and even the insects — that is, when you can feel compassion for all of creation – this sets the stage for evolving your own consciousness to higher levels. And when you can create benevolence for yourself and help to create benevolence for all other this also sets the stage for evolving your consciousness to higher levels. And all of this can allow you to increase your DNA efficiency and halt the death hormone release for a great leap in life extension.

Let an Ongoing Continuation of Your Life Unfold

You know I continually think about this idea of simply allowing my life to go on and on without the status quo ending (death) that most people expect as their probable future when they reach 80 or 90 years of age. When you begin to think this way, you begin to open up to that potential. I would like all of you to think about this and begin to let it seep in deeply. Just spend a little time in meditation or when you go about your day thinking,

"Why don't I just allow my thought patterns to evolve into seeing me, or imaging me continuing my life as it goes on and on and on, way past the 80- or 90-year current life span benchmark. Why don't I just let my thought patterns see my life journey as on-going journey without an ending and without the need for an ending."

Just begin to play with this idea and let it sink in and realize that this is a very powerful thought-mind exercise. When you begin to think like this, it naturally evolves into what can I do now that I haven't done yet that I now have time for and would like to do. Or what can I learn now that interests me that I would like to learn. Or what can I take up and become good at that I find intriguing. When you begin to think like this it may take you into a whole new career or business interest or social or community or political activity. So, you might begin to think about planning a new career. When you begin to think like this you also may think about adding new relationships to your life. A whole new world really opens up when you start thinking like this. And when you begin to think like this you absolutely do not plan on your death. Instead, you plan on an on-going life. I challenge you to begin to think like this.

Meditation to Allow an On-going Continuation

Become very calm, command your body to stillness, and go into your meditative state. Feel that your physical body is healthy and whole and in hemostatic balance. Image yourself walking on a path and feeling that your life is so wonderful, so much so, that

you say, "I love my evolving life. I love everything about my life, and about my evolving self, and I want to extend my life journey so much so that it goes on and on and on with no ending in sight." Next image a series of road signs behind you and ahead of you and the first sign way behind you reads 20 years and you have walked way past that one, and you find a sign that is at your current age and you are walking past it, and now you see the signs ahead of you and the first may read 70 years and you know you will walk past that one, and the next one reads 80 years and you know you will walk past it too, and the next reads 90 years and you know you are going to walk past that one, and the next one reads 100, and the next is 110, and 120, 130, 140, 150, 160, 170, and on. You just somehow know you are going to allow an on-going continuation of your life and walk past them all. Just savor this image for a while and decree that this is going to be the path of your life in which you are just going to allow an on-going continuation of your life to unfold.

Be Bold About Your Life Extension

If you are asked by someone at your workplace or anywhere else how long you think you are going to live, be bold about it and tell them your life extension goal. When you can do this, it solidifies a reality expectation that you ae indeed really going to do it! I have been asked several times at my workplace (once by a manager) how long I thought I was going to live and I boldly blurted out, "at least 140 to 150 years!" When you pick an age that others can accept as a possibility (even a remote possibility in their belief) it plays into your own belief system and it plays into theirs too that it is something that could be doable. And I suggest that you think about adding this to your own life extension toolbox because it will begin to create it. Indeed, be bold when it is appropriate.

What Are the Most Important Things to Go Beyond 140 to 150 Years?

To go beyond 140 to 150 years you will need to master some of the practices of the ancient masters. And work with and master some of the newer recently revealed techniques in this book that have been given. And utilize some of the new rejuvenation technologies that will become available.

1. **Utilize the Traditional Practices**
   Traditional practices include life extension affirmations, breath work and fasting, healing the death urge, deep healing, cultivating a genuine love and compassion for the earth and for all of the life forms that live upon her, and evolving into higher consciousness. Do daily life extension affirmation and go for a life span extension that works for you. Become bolder with your life extension affirmations and don't be afraid to say one to someone you often see and trust, such as a clerk in a store, "You know I have heard that the natural potential lifespan of a human is 140 to 150 years and I know that if my conviction about is strong enough I can do it even of 99% of the population doesn't think it's possible, but I know it's possible and I'm going to go for it and even longer." To say this in front of someone else you trust adds to your own sense of conviction. Refine your daily breathwork sessions and intend to bring in more oxygen and prana than before to increase your cell regeneration and intend to expel more toxins and degenerate tissues than ever before. Fast at least 1-day a week and occasionally do a 3-day fast and periodically go for even longer fasts. Restrict eating to an 8-hour window most days. Rediscover your childlike joy in living. Learn to be playful. Learn to develop a knowledge base of living continually is a state of contentment and acknowledge the freedom from disease that this brings you. Work on all of these.

2. **Incorporate the Modern Practices**
   Modern practices include learning how to live without fearing disease. Ascertain what it means to go through life without fearing disease. Develop the consciousness that knows what is out of balance and knows how to rebalance it. Move to a diet that supports life extension. Maintaining an adequate fitness level through exercise and yoga. Become

able to heal deeply by restructuring your emotional body and your mental body such that your emotions always mirror contentment and your thoughts are carefully formulated so that they are always of a non-condemning nature with the goals of the six perfections and nine deep healers in mind.

3. **Develop Higher Consciousness**
    What is attaining higher consciousness? It is having compassion for all life and wanting to see all life happy and fulfilled in their life journey. It is having higher thought consciousness where all thoughts of strife, struggle, conflict, brute force, resentments, ill will, etc. are eliminated. It is expecting only good things to happen. It is expecting benevolence. It is always seeking to keep the peace through peaceful non-violent means. It is seeking to have your primal energy field and your body's DNA vibrating in a coherent manner. It is continually developing the higher mental abilities (telepathy) and the psychic abilities (astral projection, thought projection, bilocation, etc.) Start cultivating higher consciousness thoughts and emotions. Begin to develop your genius self. Begin to think of becoming a genius who has amazing knowledge in a wide variety of fields and subjects. Become a genius who is like a sponge able to absorb an amazing amount of wisdom.

4. **Add the Higher Dimensional Spiritual Technologies**
    Modern practices also include: all of the energy exercises and meditations in this book, such as shimmering, soul loss retrieval, increasing your DNA efficiency, stopping the death hormone release, releasing your bias to expect bad things, doing your daily affirmations, doing your future human meditations, and doing the mind-power youthing and rejuvenation meditation.

5. **Cultivate Perfection and Purification**
    Life extension students should come to know the importance of perfecting the physical body, the emotional body, the

mental body, and the spirit body or soul. Many practices in both the physical arena and in higher dimensional realms have been outlined and the intermediate life extension student is asked to begin to cultivate perfection of the physical body form that the consciousness occupies, and to purify the thoughts andemotions to those of the higher consciousness of benevolence.

It's Actually Hard Work to Age Yourself

Yes, it is. It's hard work to age yourself. Think about it. To age yourself you have to constantly create ego-driven thoughts of resentment, envy, dissatisfaction with life, irritation with others, general unhappiness, etc., etc., etc. It is hard work to do all that. Stop working so hard. Relax into a general contentment with the way things are. Don't fret over what you don't have. Joy in the small things in life. Learn to be calm. Create joyful relationships with others. Over time you will come to realize that it's actually easier and less work to simply extend your life. You will learn that it's less work to let your life move into an on-going pleasant journey that will be called life extension. So, stop working so hard to age yourself!

Suggestions for the Life Extension Seeker

The life extension aspirant is encouraged to read this chapter several times and do the exercise for halting the death hormone release and for increasing your DNA efficiency several times over the next three months. The life extension aspirant is challenged to work with and incorporate the affirmations below.

Intermediate Life Extension Affirmations

1. As a life extender, I am going to go for an extended life span of al least 200 years. I know that even if 99% of the population does not think it is possible, I know that if my conviction is strong enough, I can do it no matter what anyone thinks. And I decree that my conviction IS strong enough and I AM going to do it!

2. As a life extender, I am invoking the power of my mind to change my beliefs and thought patterns so that my expanded beliefs, thoughts and expectations allow me to go for a greater than 200-year life span, and I intend to be quietly fanatical about it! Yes, I am a quiet life extension fanatic!

3. I, as a life extender, intend to let it seep in deeply that my body is designed to let me live over 300 hundred years, not just a mere 80 to 100. Yes, yes!

4. I am allowing my life extension affirmations to go deeper and deeper and really sink in. I plan on adding everything that will help them manifest my decree to extend my life to 200 years and beyond. I understand that this also means I will let go of everything that will stop me from reaching this goal.

5. I am stopping the aging clock and the death hormone release by working with the energy exercise meditation to instruct my primal energy field, and all of my body's cells, and my whole body to stop this. Indeed, I will master this!

6. I am working on increasing the efficiency of my DNA through intention, visualization, energy exercises, meditation, and by developing higher consciousness. Indeed, I will master this!

7. I am a reality bender. I can bend my reality such that the outcome is always good for me. I intend to bend my reality into the life of a life extender. Yes, yes!

8. I, as a life extender, know that all illness and degeneration can be healed and on a routine basis I work with what my body needs most to keep it in a balanced and healed state, and to keep it looking like a youthful mature person.

9. I am developing the ability to move forward in life without fearing disease. Oh yes! I am, indeed!

10. I am aware that all disease offers a cleansing opportunity, and that after it has run its course, I know I will feel better because of the elimination of toxins that the disease will have removed. Yes!

11. I am healing deeply by working with the six perfections. Yes!

12. I am deeply healing by working with the nine deep healers. Yes!

13. I, as a life extender, am learning to cultivate contentment, neutrality, and equanimity, indeed!

14. I know that part of life extension is to become a kinder and more loving person and I continually work on becoming a kinder and more loving person.

15. I know that the twelve universal laws hold much wisdom for life extension and I intend to learn and work with and incorporate the wisdom of the twelve universal laws.

16. I, as a life extender, intend to wean myself away from early planned death that is continually bombarded at us from Medicare, life insurance, funeral homes and the like. I refuse to plan for my death by not getting involved in any of this. I plan on extending my life and that is all there is to it!

17. I, as a life extender, know that my life is about having an important mission and there are plenty of things that need to change to make our word a better place, and I intend to choose the most meaningful and important of these needed purposes that I resonate to, and I intend to get involved with them to help make the needed changes happen.

18. I, as a life extender, in an on-going basis intend to gravitate to a diet more suited to life extension.

19. I, as a life extender, in an on-going basis intend to gravitate towards better and better removal of toxins and I intend to avoid toxins in food and drink.

20. I, as a life extender, in an on-going basis intend to gravitate towards better and better control of my thoughts and my emotions so that my thoughts and emotions are always centered on what's best for the whole.

21. I, as a life extender, am going to add fasting. I will do either Intermittent Fasting, or the 1-day a week fast, and occasionally I will do longer fasts as is appropriate for my life extension in an on-going basis.

22. I, as a life extender, will do daily breathwork sessions as appropriate for my life extension in an on-going basis.

Physical, emotional and mental perfection and deep healing are prerequisites for immortality.

Masters, such as Jesus, have always said, "What I can do, you can [learn to] do also."

Part 3

Advanced Life Extension Practices

CHAPTER 9
The Interdimensional Connection

Much new information has been revealed in recent year to help humanity live longer and some of it goes beyond the third dimensional realm. Many higher dimensional processes and practices will not only help you live longer, but will also greatly increase your psychic abilities. And they will increase your health by not allowing any disease to develop. Some of these higher dimensional spiritual technologies include shimmering your auric field, retrieving your lost soul fragments, and assimilating higher dimensional knowledge of your DNA, and your chakra, and kundalini systems, and your soul's connection to your lower personality.

Shimmering

It is important to look at the spiritual practice called shimmering. It is related to your personal and planetary evolution. And it can set up a needed protection for your auric field. Shimmering is considered to be one of the main spiritual technologies and it can be described as a rapid increase in the pulse rate of your aura. Your aura is a part of your primal energy field and it has a pulse rate, just as your circulation system pulses in rhythm with your heartbeat. The pulse of your aura can reach very high frequencies. In fact, the higher the pulse of your aura, the greater your spiritual awareness and your spiritual energy becomes and this will increase your psychic abilities dramatically. It is interesting to note that there is a vibrational curtain that separates the 3rd dimension from the 5th dimension and the reason for this curtain is to keep people of the lower vibrations of hate and jealousy, and those who want to dominate and control others out of the 5th dimension. The practice of shimmering allows you to increase the speed of your aura and go through the veil and curtain between the 3rd and 5th dimensions. Shimmering does require some basic observation of the human aura because it requires some conceptualization and understanding of the aura.

One way to work with shimmering is to think of your aura or auric field as a giant egg. This egg shape can be thought of as the optimal shape of the human aura. You can intuit and visualize that the outer edge of your aura has a line that goes around the aura energy field and that this line forms the shape of your aura. When doing aura shimmering see if you can notice if there are any holes or indentations or parasitic attachments in it. Mentally drawing a line that goes around your aura can fill in these holes and stop energy leakages and that is important because life force energy that leaks out ages you. The most common reason that people can have holes in their aura is due to traumatic events. Especially from posttraumatic stress and war trauma. Parasitic attachments are hooks or tentacles from other people and through these hooks they can take away your energy. Mentally drawing a line (you can make the line green, blue or purple or any color) around your aura is one way to become aware of them. In addition, the line gives you a focal pattern for beginning to pulse your aura. When you increase the speed of your aura, it becomes much easier to repair it. In fact, lower parasitic tentacles and lower parasitic attachments cannot stick, stay, or be parasitically attached to an aura that pulses and vibrates at a higher speed. When a person pulses or vibrates their aura at a high speed there can be an amazing and miraculous healing to their aura. Another very valuable thing about shimmering or accelerating your aura pulse rate is that many illnesses can be healed. Some illness come from holes or cracks or fissures in your aura, and they cause energy leakages. In fact, air borne pathogens must travel through your aura to get to your body and vibrating your aura at high speeds more easily repels them. Indeed, there are many, many benefits to shimmering.

Let us now visualize that the line around the outer edge of your aura has a deep or bright purple color of a very solid nature. Now, for the purposes of shimmering exercises you can visualize that your aura extends outward from your skin about 8 inches. Experts can project their aura out 40-50-60 inches from the body but for our work here in talking about shimmering, it is recommended that the length you work with is 8 inches from your body which will provide maximum benefit for your shimmering. Start with becoming aware of your existing aura pulse speed. This is similar to becoming aware of your breathing cycle rate. In breathwork classes, an instructor may say, "Become aware of your breathing without changing it in any way." It is the same with aura work. Become aware of your aura and its present pulse rate. Start by chanting a tone to a rhythm that you should try match in pulsing your aura to it. The tone might be a slow: ta ta ta ta ta ta ta ta ta ta ta, at maybe 1 count per second for two to three minutes. By making this tone, you can try to match your aura pule rate to it. Then you can increase the speed of the tone to a faster: ta ta ta ta ta ta ta ta ta, to 2 counts per second, and keep up this pace for another 2-3 minutes. Then increase it again to: tatatatatatatatata, to 3 counts per second for 2-3 minutes. You should now sense your energy field and your aura pulsing much faster. In shimmering, you expand and contract the size of your aura cosmic egg to match your shimmering speed – your auric field cosmic egg expands and contracts, expands and contracts, expands and contracts.

When you become adept at this and you are able to shimmer your aura at a very fast pulse rate, you will begin to flicker or shimmer. That means that you are going in and out of physical awareness and others observing you will would see your energy flicker which means it would go in and out and seem to go into another realm. There are also sacred tones and sounds that you should use before you shimmer. The Chinese Taoist tone of 'huuuuhhh' and 'haaah' are very effective and should be used. You should practice shimmering in a space you designate as a sacred space. You should practice shimmering at a time you designate as sacred. You can use crystals and special stones to assist you in increasing and holding your vibrational frequency. Shimmering protects the energy field around you which is compromised by many energy bombardments daily.

A Shimmering Exercise

Direct your aura to assume the shape of a giant egg (the cosmic egg). The shape is like a giant chicken egg but it surrounds your body eight inches out from your skin and your aura just fits inside. Next, verbalize the Chinese Taoist tones of 'huuuuhhh' and 'haaah' before starting this shimmering exercise. Now, sense your cosmic egg aura and match its expansion-contraction pulse rate to the following slow tone at one count per second: ta ta ta ta ta ta ta ta ta ta ta, for two or three minutes. Next, double the speed of the tone to: ta ta ta ta ta ta ta ta ta, to two counts per second for 2-3 minutes. Now increase it again: tatatatatatatatata, to three counts per second for 2-3 minutes. You should be able to sense your energy field and your aura pulsing much faster now.

Water Shimmering

Whenever you are near water, it is a good idea to take a moment to be with the water especially if the sun shines and flickers and seems to shimmer on it. Breathe into this moment and say huuuuhhh' and 'haaah' before starting this shimmering and shimmer with the water, tatatattatatatata. See your body shimmering with light. This raises your vibration quickly, rejuvenating your body's organs. It helps restore flow to your meridians points, your circulatory system and your body's organs.

At this stage we are still at a primitive level in protecting our energy fields. Shimmering can help open what is called the assemblage point (as termed by native shamans) on your body and this is a key to partly lifting the third dimensional veil. When you begin to shimmer and increase the speed of your aura you will have major increases in all of your spiritual psychic abilities. Your ability to use your 3rd eye will increase dramatically. Your ability to be telepathic will increase. Your ability to heal will increase too. And ultimately your ability to thought-project will increase. You should also know that at the higher speeds of your aura, where you thought-project place your aura is where your physical body follows. At lower speeds, of course, where your body goes is where your aura goes. All of this is preparatory to thought-projecting yourself into the 5th dimension, but that is another subject altogether.

Soul Fragmentation

Have you ever heard of soul fragmentation?
If an organ loses some energy of the soul
It dries up – you age – this takes a physical toll.
Soul fragmentation causes organ degeneration.

Whenever you are facing trauma or feeling real fear
A small bit of your soul fragments off and flies away.
Soul vibration is much higher than fear, it cannot stay
Near when fear is here – a fragment will fly away.

Where does it go? Into nature is where it goes.
Tree, bushes, ground, grasses, especially water
Are where it goes – a parent, son or daughter
Like being near water where soul energy flows.

Thousands of soul fragmentations have happened to you
But energy exercises exist for you – you are your body's boss
To recover and retrieve some of your soul fragmentation loss.
Then lost abilities from soul loss can be returned back to you.

Soul Loss and Soul Retrieval

Soul fragmentation happens all throughout life and soul loss affects the aging mechanism in all of the organs and tissues of your body, bloodstream, bones and skin. If the vitality of your soul leaves your organs they will slowly dry up. But if you are able to maintain your organs in the high-vibrational frequency of your divine soul, you will have more light within and then your organs will not age. When your organs do not age your body does not age. A human body is designed to live 300 to 900 years, but soul loss is one of important things that cuts your longevity far short of this. Many of the yoga gurus of yesteryear have actually demonstrated this immortality, and preserving the life force energy has always been one of their revered and sacred practices. They have always said that each person is born with a certain amount of 'soul essence' and that preventing the loss of some of this soul essence was an important part of their immortality practices. In their day they used bandas or postures to prevent soul loss. In our day, other spiritual technologies have been revealed to us to help humans learn soul loss recovery retrieval techniques. And other practices have been given to help us add more life force energy.

When you ask, "Why do people age?" one of the more important (and unrecognized) reasons is because of the depletion of the life force energy due to soul fragmentation. When soul fragmentation occurs, your aura collapses, and holes, cracks and fissures appear in it, and then the chi or life force energy can seep out of these holes, cracks and fissures and then you age. An example of this is found in humans who have lived very hard and harsh lives fraught with continual struggle that cause constant soul fragmentation and you can tell the aging caused by this in their faces.

So, what exactly is it that causes soul fragmentation to happen and when does it occur? Soul fragmentation can occur on a daily basis and people are never even aware that it happens. Whenever excessive fear occurs, part of the soul fragments off because your high frequency soul energy cannot handle this fear energy low vibration. And when this soul fragmentation occurs, a small part of your soul that contains the gifts and abilities that you have, leaves you. Some of the native peoples know this and tribal shamans may perform a soul retrieval ceremony for tribal members who have had an experience that put great fear in their hearts—maybe they had a fearful encounter with a dangerous animal, or they might have been in a battle where they were required to kill or feared that they would be killed.

Soul fragmentation happens throughout life. Soul fragmentation happens even in the mother's womb before birth, and the mother and father's thoughts and emotional states affect the unborn child greatly. Conventional soul fragmentation starts about ten days before birth when the baby instinctively knows it must leave the comfort and safety of the womb and enter the hostile and dense world. Another soul fragmentation happens when the baby knows it must pass through the dark birth canal. The third fragmentation takes place when the baby is born and it must switch to breathing air which is confusing and causes great fear and that causes great soul loss. A cesarean section causes soul loss for the mother and the baby. A premature birth where the baby is taken away from the mother causes tremendous soul loss for the baby which negatively affect the mental, emotional, spiritual, and auric bodies throughout life. Natural birth is best. Between 2 and 3 years old, children recognize people from past lives and this sometimes brings up fear from bad experiences they had and soul loss happens. From 4½ to 12, personality is formed and children most often hear "no" from their parents, grandparents and teachers and they are often disappointed in not getting what they want and this depletes their energy fields. From 12 to 17, their bodies change hormonally causing confusion and often causes soul fragmentation. When early puppy love pairs break up there is great hurt and soul loss. From 16 to 21 there is pressure to conform to peer groups and if there is pressure to fit in along with bulling, and not being taken seriously, and being rejected by a peer group or a friend, this causes loss of personal power and results in soul fragmentation.

You may have heard of a 10-year-old child who was severely bullied and then commits suicide. In such a case there was great soul loss. After 21, people enter the workplace and sometimes face hostile environments with great peer pressure to perform, conform, and please the boss and this causes soul fragmentation. At 24 people date more seriously and breakups can lead to soul loss. From the beginning of life to around 30, more than 5,000 soul fragmentations happen to the average person. Each one causes your aura to collapse, and holes and cracks to appear in it, and then your chi or life force energy seeps out through these holes, cracks and fissures, even though you are not aware of it.

So again, why do people age? One of the most unrecognized but important factors is the depletion of life force chi energy because of soul fragmentation. And if you look at those who have lived hard lives with continuous struggle, you will see aging in their faces, and you can connect this to the soul loss they have suffered. And a great many soul fragmentations have happened by ages 60 through 70—probably over 10,000 for the average person, and that is when aging and organ degeneration really becomes pronounced! It is important to know that soul fragmentation happens all throughout life and this soul loss causes your aura to collapse, and holes and cracks to develop in it through which your chi or life force energy seeps out. And since your soul is in your entire body, soul loss affects the aging mechanism in all of the organs and tissues of your body, bloodstream, bones and skin. If the vitality of your soul leaves your organs they will slowly dry up and then age. But if you are able to maintain your organs in the high-vibrational frequency – we will say it again, in the high vibration of your divine soul then you will have more light within you, and your organs will not age. When your organs do not age, your body will not age. It needs to be re-emphasized that your body was designed to live over 300 to 900 years, and preventing soul fragmentation is an important aspect of this.

Many yoga masters of immortality have shown this – have lived hundreds of years and proven it, and demonstrated it, and one of their tenets has always been to keep their life force energy or chi and prevent it from fragmenting and seeping out. Now, let us ask where do your soul fragments go when they are lost, and whether or not your soul fragments can be retrieved and brought back to you. Your lost soul fragments go into nature. They go into the trees and the plants and the water. When you are near water, you feel good because you feel the collective soul fragment energy of many people. When some of your soul parts are reconnected to you, you feel uplifted as you are able to feel more of your soul life force energy. Can you recollect your soul fragments? The answer is, yes you can. So, let us examine now some of the techniques and methods for retrieving and reclaiming your missing soul fragments. There are several of these techniques. And there are masters and angles who can assist humans in collecting and retrieving their soul fragments including Sananda (Jesus), Buddha, Archangel Michael and many, many others.

A good technique to start working with this is to call on them to help you retrieve your soul fragments. Simply call forth the cohabitation energy of the masters and the angles and your spirit guides twice daily—early in the morning and when you go sleep. And ask them to assist you to recover your lost soul fragments before you start a visualization-meditation exercise to do this. They can be helpful in retrieving soul loss from many types of traumas, and the list is a long one including: not feeling worthy or good enough, fearing man or God, pre-birth soul loss, soul loss due to your country of birth, grief from death or illness or surgery, grief or anger over a broken heart in a relationship, from deep disappointment in life, from spiritual disappointment, from lost Atlantis soul fragments, etc. Be thankful for the help these beings offer to help recover soul loss. Here are some soul loss recovery exercises you can use to recover your own soul loss.

Exercises to Recover Soul Loss

Retrieve Soul Loss Caused by 'Disappointment'

Go outdoors where you will not be disturbed and imagine or create an image of a spiral of light next to you that is going up from the earth up to the universe. Ask for and feel the presence of a higher beings who will work with you to help retrieve some of your lost soul fragments. With the higher being standing next to you (perhaps an angle, archangel, Sananada or an ascended master) breathe into this image, this visualization, and become one with the spiral of light and the higher being. Ask for help in retrieving your lost soul fragments due to disappointment. Do this periodically for 3 days. Sense soul fragments returning to you.

Retrieve Soul Loss Caused by 'Fear'

Do this exercise when you feel you have lost some of your life force chi energy and it has gone into the ground from your feeling fear or stress. Bring in your spirit team (your spirit guides, and an angle or archangel or ascended master) and before starting ask for help to retrieve some of your lost soul fragment energy. Find a quiet place and using a stick, scrie a big circle around you, then draw a pyramid inside the circle and stand in the middle and breathe from the ground to reclaim your soul fragment energy that has gone into the ground, trees, water, and the other elements. Breathe this energy back into you for three to five minutes. You can also make the circle and pyramid with a string of rocks, or branches or pinecones or sand or any other item from nature.

Retrieve Soul Loss from 'Intense Emotions'

During full moons is a good time for you to recover some soul fragmented energy that was lost by intense emotional issues. The moon supports emotional well-being inside you and it is the ruler of water. Soul fragmentation reduces the light within the water in your body so that less spiritual light can reside within you. Working with the moon, especially the full moon, can replenish this spiritual light energy. You can light a candle and have a white flower or white cloth in both palms. Bring in your spirit team. Meditate on the moon and imagine a beautiful light from the moon is entering your thirty-third chakra all the way down to your soul star chakra beneath your feet. And then ask that the soul fragments that you have lost due to intense emotional issues become returned to you.

Retrieve Soul Fragments Using Sound

Certain ancient sounds and mudras can call forth fragmented parts of the soul because they can put your human body in resonance with the vibrational frequency of the earth. These sounds come from ancient languages that have a high frequency and are calibrated with the frequency of earth and your body and they bring you into instant healing energy. "Aum...aum...aum...aum...aum," the Sanskrit sound, "Aum," (not Om) opens meridians, earth's and yours, and when you tone this sound for several minutes a flow of energy comes into you. "Aurr...aurrr...aurrr...aurrr" The Hebrew sound, "Aurr," when said with a mudra connects your higher aspects to solar, universal and multidimensional levels and this lets you download higher frequencies from your oversoul into your earth reality. Make the hand position or mudra by pointing with the index finger and then wrapping the middle finger around it, and then touch the other two fingers to the thumb. Then move this hand position between your mouth and third eye, and then say, "Aurrr aurr," and then bring in your spirit team and ask for help in retrieving some of your lost soul fragments from the earth and from higher solar, universal and multidimensional levels.

Exercises to Add Chi (Life Force) Energy

Adding Chi Energy

Imagine that a beautiful sphere of golden-white light is covering you. And imagine that you are a part of this golden-white light and that the sphere and you are shimmering (pulsing with light) like a strobe light at an ever-increasing rate: ta-ta-ta...pulsing, pulsing, pulsing. Image that you and the sphere of golden-white light are shimmering faster and faster and faster at a very high pulse rate. Sense being infused with chi energy. Do this for 3-5 minutes.

Infusing Yourself with Chi

Create an image of a golden ball pulsing with light. Watch it pulse, and visualize the pulsing light flooding into you with every pulse. Visualize every part of your body being infused with this pulsing light, pulsing, pulsing, pulsing. Imagine that your body's vital organs are being infused and energized by the golden light from this golden ball. This will help you regain your personal power so that you feel you are the one in charge of your body and all of its organs, glands, tissues and structures so that you can instruct them to stop aging and to youth. Do this for 3-5 minutes.

Massage to Remove Trauma and Add Chi

Massage is a time-honored way to release past life trauma and allow life force energy to reoccupy that space. People all over the world instinctively do massage. When mothers massage their newborn babies it sends energy into the baby's organs to supplement lost soul fragments. In adults, deep massage can bring to the surface past life traumas and release them and this allows life force chi energy to once again re-enter and occupy that space that was blocked by the negative energy.

Remove Soul Attachments

Soul attachment may cause the fears, insecurities, belief systems and thought patterns of those whose soul fragments are attached to you to influence your own personality self and this can interfere with your own spiritual development. It is important to free yourself from this and detach these unwanted fragments. You must ask and speak out loud that these fragments be disconnected. You will not know which soul fragments are attached to you or which soul part has fragmented and left. Simply asking for the unwanted soul fragment to leave is enough. Asking for the wanted missing fragment to return is enough. You don't need to know all the details.

Auric Field Maintenance

Auric maintenance should be done on a daily basis by doing the cosmic egg, shimmering, and aura smoothing. Another powerful spiritual practice to bring higher frequencies to yourself is to use cohabitation which is joining with the higher frequencies of your guides, masters, and angles. You will feel stronger in your organs as you raise your vibrations and it is to be noted that your aura interacts with higher frequencies. Dense energy that you may have picked up cannot stay in your auric field because it will dissolve in the higher frequencies of your guides, the masters and the angles. So, it is a very good idea to practice using cohabitation by joining with the higher frequencies of your guides, the masters and the angles. Simply call forth the cohabitation energy of your guides, the masters and the angles twice daily—early in the morning and when you go sleep. Along with auric maintenance on a daily basis you should work with reclaiming your soul fragmentation energy to maintain higher frequencies and stop aging. This process may take a while, but you will eventually know that you have integrated a large part of yourself and brought back many of your lost soul parts and original energy.

Signs of Retrieved and Restored Soul Fragments

When you have successfully collected and integrated lost soul fragments you will be surprised and pleased to discover that new talents and abilities that you never had before will start to come out. They could be simple or profound. You will also start to trust and believe in yourself more and more and not need validation from others as much. After integrating Shakipat energies (the transmission of spiritual energy upon one person by another consciousness), you might start to channel and bring in sound codes, light languages, and sacred geometry. When this happens, you have replenished the higher frequencies from the galaxies and the masters which naturally opens your inherent and latent abilities.

Higher Knowledge, Part 1

Your DNA Has 12 Layers

Indeed, the increasing lifespan among humans will be partly due to the greater knowledge of the higher dimensional aspects of your body. Your whole body and many of its parts have higher dimensional aspects, especially your DNA. When science looks at DNA it only sees the first layer which is the only physical layer, and science only sees the familiar double helix. But there are actually twelve layers to your DNA, and the other eleven are interdimensional. Each layer has a meaning and a purpose and several layers work together as a team. Your soul is in one of the interdimensional DNA layers. The twelfth layer is called the God layer, and it is your connection to God. When you learn this, you can begin to understand that, "You are made in the image of God," actually means, "You are made in the image of benevolent love," for that is what God is. When you know, you are connected to God and benevolent love through your DNA, you can actually begin to allow a life of benevolence to unfold for yourself, and this will increase your longevity.

Your Aura and Kundalini Have 7 Layers

When you learn that your aura and your kundalini energy are each composed of seven layers, and that each layer is connected to one of your chakras, and that all of your seven major chakras are connected to each other through the gossamer interdimensional threads of your 144,000 meridian system, and that each chakra is connected to one of your endocrine glands, and that these directly affect your physical body—when you learn all this and know all of this you have information to help you live longer. Your attitude and mood are also very important for both your aura and your chakras. The higher your vibration, the more you live in joy and thanksgiving and appreciation, the more your aura becomes a transmuting system and transmutes low vibration energy and issues high vibration energy—and this is very healing and it helps your longevity. If say, you are betrayed, but you are already in a high vibrational place of thankfulness then your aura can transmute the low vibrational energy of the betrayal so your aura can be a protective energy field – it can transmute low vibrational energy. If you can stay in the depth of your heart so that your vibration raises when you breathe out and releases the anger or fear or even hatred of the betrayal—that energy does not go out into the world as hatred, anger or fear. Instead, it passes into your aura where it is transmuted according to your vibration of the moment and then out into the world. This energizes your aura which in turn downloads into your chakras which in turn brings more energy into your endocrine system and this in turn brings more energy into your entire physical body and help you live longer.

Fear Closes Your Chakras

Also, it is important to know that the prana or life force energy which along with the food you eat is what fuels your body. And actually, you should know that your body is fueled more by the incoming prana than it is by the food that you eat. And your body takes prana in through your breath, and through your chakras (which are spinning energy vortexes) when they are open, and they are only open when you are living in joy and thanksgiving and appreciation. But your chakras are closed when you are in fear. And so, this is another reason why maintaining the higher spectrum of thoughts and emotions is part of attaining higher consciousness.

Your Physical Body Is an Entity unto Itself

Another thing to learn is that your physical body is a being unto itself that you live within. Your physical body is an entity in and of itself and it would like to live forever. Your physical body wants you to keep it whole and healthy. It does not want to die – it enjoys life. It needs exercise, it needs nutrition, and it also needs to experience joy.

Higher Knowledge, Part 2

Your Triangle of Beingness

Indeed, the increasing lifespan among humans will be partly due to the greater knowledge of the higher dimensional aspects of your body. The three parts of the triangle of beingness for a human play very important roles in developing the ability to move forward without fearing disease. There are three parts to your personality construct or your beingness. The three parts are: the physical, the mental, and the emotional. And each of these is encased within its own sheath. The first sheath is your physical body and is what you are most familiar with and it must always be kept in a good state of physical health. Good nutrition and moderate exercise are always important for this.

The second sheath of your triangle of beingness is not so well known or understood, but it has a major effect on your health. It is your aetheric body and it is a body sheath that is made of a thickened shell of the aether which envelopes your body and extends out about one sixteenth of an inch from the skin. This sheath actually forms quite a good barrier against microbes and you might have noticed that you are more susceptible for getting an infection when you suffer a cut that breaches both your skin and your aetheric sheath. Your aetheric body sheath or web is also comprised of your major and minor chakras and your vast 144,000 energy meridian grid network. One of the most important things about your aetheric body sheath is that it is directly connected to your thoughts. It actually responds to and reflects your thoughts. That is why older people who constantly think they are getting older and older actually create it because their aetheric sheath begins to conform to the oldness of the thought image that is constantly being projected to it, and in about nine months, this aetheric sheath old-body-image thought-form actually downloads into the physical body and from there it makes the physical body older. That is why the masters always cultivate higher thought images of themselves as youthful looking older mature people. Your mental body must be trained to maintain preponderant thought patterns of yourself in health and as a person in mature prime of life if that is the case. As you develop this ability you may be able to reach a state where you can tell whether or not all of your physical bodily systems are all in balance or not and working properly or not. This involves developing knowledge of when you have a mental energy flow blockage, and then being able to release that blockage so that your body's energy flow and nutrient flow and waste removal and all other body systems are balanced and in hemostasis. Your aetheric body sheath is directly connected to the second triangle of beingness which is your mental body. These three parts of the triangle of beingness always need to be kept in a state of balance such that one does not dominate the other. If the mental side dominates the personality complex this sets up conditions for the affliction of dementia to manifest. Dementia sufferers over mentalize and do not allow their emotional or physical sides full expression.

The third sheath is your astral body. Your astral body sheath is sometimes called your dream body because it is what you see when you see yourself in your dreams. Your astral body was the vehicle that your personality consciousness inhabited during your incarnational birth, and your astral vehicle is what your personality consciousness will inhabit when it leaves your physical body after your life is finally over. Your astral body sheath is a direct replica of your physical body, organ for organ, gland for gland, bone for bone, tissue for tissue, but it is made of a much finer substance. Those who have lost a limb, but say that they can see and feel a ghost limb, are actually seeing and feeling their astral limb counterpart which is still there. Your astral body is actually the seat of, or the origin of, your emotions. And indulging in chronic negative emotions directly affects the health of your astral body which again in about nine months downloads the damage into your physical body. Indulging in lower spectrum emotions such as suffering, grief, hatred, pettiness, greed, jealousy, low self-worth, fear, panic, worry, anger, rage, resentment, regret, and aggression will all take a toll on the health of your astral body and from there it will eventually affect your physical health. What directly affects the health of your astral body in a positive way are the higher spectrum emotions including feelings of empowerment, joy, bliss, reverence, peace, love, empathy, and well-being. It is important to develop the skill of living in the higher emotions, and it is important to learn to become slow to anger. Cultivating the six perfections and the nine healers are important steps in this direction. Again, the three parts of the triangle of beingness need to be kept in a state of balance such that one does not dominate the other. If the emotional side dominates the personality complex, this sets up conditions for raging out of control and this can, and often does result in heart disease and, of course, in damaging conflicts with others. Master teachers in the past have pointedly said that disease or debilitation first occurs in your aetheric body or in your astral body, and from there it gradually infiltrates into your physical vessel.

Communication Between Your Personality Complex and Your Soul

The Biblical Jacob was given a dream in which he was shown two ladders climbing to sky and there were angles in single file walking up one ladder and angles in single file walking down the other ladder. While many interpretations have been given for this, one meaning is that it symbolized the constant two-way flow of communication and energy from your lower personality complex to your higher self or soul and then back again. Indeed, this two-way flow is an integral part of understanding the higher dimensional connection of your lower personality complex to your higher self and soul complex. New experiences from your current life flows up to your soul, and wisdom from all of your past lives flows down from your soul to your personality complex as wisdom you can use to make decisions with.

Also, if some part of your lower body has a short-fall of energy, your soul can and often does send energy to the part that needs it. Sometimes this soul energy saves a human life by providing enough energy the body can use to overcome an illness as in miracle healings. Your soul communicates to you through your emotional and your mental bodies. The emotional communications from your soul come through your heart center, and the mental communications from your soul come through your pineal gland, which connects to the higher vibrational part of your brain called the sacred mind. When the communication and connection is strong, your physical body reaps the rewards by way of better health and vitality as well as a deeper connection with your primal energy field. And the communication and connection will always be strong when you are in contentment and are not in fear. And as you tap into the higher frequencies of divine wisdom, brilliant ideas will pour forth from the higher planes of intuition. Your soul and the souls of eight other humans (totaling nine) are all connected to an oversoul, and this oversoul (along with eight other oversouls) is connected a higher oversoul and this goes on and on until it eventually reaches the Creator.

Metabolizing light (prana) is an important and intricate process that is very necessary for your well-being. It could be said that humans have been on a starvation diet of half half-spectrum God light. Your trillions of cells must relearn how to recognize and utilize this higher vibrational light that is now coming in as a vital energy source, and when you start attaining and attuning to higher consciousness you naturally begin to do this. The new reality of the senses or physical body consciousness when you begin to evolve into higher consciousness is that when you are in the flow of spirit, and happy, and contented, you exist very lightly in your body, often with no pain or discomfort at all, and you may experience some diminished bodily sensations, except within the deep sacred heart area where you will gradually begin to feel a loving bliss and joy as they blaze forth. And more and more often, you will experience a great sense of well-being, harmony and peace.

Your Sacred Mind and your Soul's Galactic Connection

Spiritual developed human beings are those who have developed their superconscious abilities enough so that they may begin to draw on the wealth of information stored in their sacred minds. Eventually earth humans will gain the ability to draw forth inspiration and advanced information from the higher dimensions via the many aspects of their soul selves which are scattered throughout this galaxy. Your superconscious mind and your higher self are your links to the higher spiritual realms. At first, you may begin to get flashes of information and inspiration from your intuitive abilities and during meditation. The powers of your mind will be greatly enhanced as an aspirant on the path of becoming more proficient and comfortable in using the higher frequency patterns of your sacred mind. As a result of tapping into those higher frequency realms of your brain structure, a good portion of your memory of past events will begin to fade away, and this will allow you to move out of the realm of instinctive mind and past life trauma into the realm of the higher mind and benevolent creation.

Suggestions for the Life Extension Student

The life extension student is invited to do all of the exercises in this chapter many times. When you can cognate this information, it can help you move into life extension. Eventually, when you really become a master at being able to utilize this knowledge you can co-create a life span that will join with those of the human galactic brotherhood.

Perfection Means Attaining Mastery of Spiritual Technology

CHAPTER 10
Rejuvenation

It is important to understand that any new worldwide sweeping change faces obstacles and resistance and the leap into great life extension is no exception. Many established industries, religious belief systems, and ways of life will need to change to incorporate human life spans that are much, much longer than they ae now: at first twice as long, and then a few generations later, three times as long, and it is expected that there will be resistance to this change. Life insurance policies will need to change, retirement pensions will need to be updated, changes will need to happen throughout the current existing human complex social, cultural, industrial, governmental and religious organizations to accommodate the greatly increased life spans and even at this very early stage this life extension movement is already creating substantial resistance against it. There are said to be three stages involved in any new world-wide sweeping change before it is finally accepted.

Stage 1 – It is ridiculed and denied as impossible and foolhardy

Stage 2 – It is attacked and condemned as risky and unacceptable

Stage 3 – It is finally accepted and embraced as a given

However, that said, I would like to relate a dream communication during the 2020 Christmas and New Year's Holidays. The following quote from a published article kept surfacing in my mind over the course of several days, "Atlantis rejuvenation was a complex process that enabled a complete rebooting of the cells and organs of the body, and in being a complex process [or group of processes] it led to very long lifespans of over 1,000 years!" The quote continued and said that those who were allowed to use the complex technologies and processes were capable of extremely long, life spans, both through the rejuvenation of mind-thought-power and through the use of the many technologies that had been created: The Temple of Rejuvenation, Radon Health spas, the twelve-foot-high phi-angle faceted crystals containing trace amounts of gold, and a special living green phosphoric mineral called the 'philosopher's stone'. But the main thing that struck me about this was the comment that Atlantis Rejuvenation was complex and it consisted of many anti-aging devices, processes, systems and techniques. It was not just one process. The Temple of Rejuvenation was said to be a cornerstone process. But there were other methods, and among them were the radon gas radiation treatments. As I kept deeply pondering all of this for several days, especially the radon gas rejuvenation treatments, seemingly out of the blue during sleep I was given a dream, and in the dream, I saw myself looking for the slightly radioactive mineral thorium, and then I heard voice in my head very plainly say, "Why not go for 230 years [instead of only 200 years] by adding the slightly radioactive radon gas treatments?"

To me this clearly says that if you add radon radiation treatments, the results can be so beneficial that another 30 more years of life extension becomes possible! And so, the dream seemed to indicate that these life extension treatments and processes and technologies are all additive. Each new treatment or process or teaching that you master can increase the number of years that you can extend your life. First, we will first look at treatments and technologies currently available from the external science that can assist you in rejuvenating your body. Then we will look at age reversal technologies that are in the works and being developed for rejuvenation. And last, we will present some of the new revelations from the internal science for youthing your body.

Rejuvenation through External Science

The momentum in the bio-tech medical science community for creating age reversal and rejuvenation technologies is rapidly gaining a strong foothold on the world stage. Many new hi-tech and bio-tech startups, and a few well-established health giants, are racing to develop anti-aging and age reversal technical modalities and interventions. As of 2022, there are three promising technologies under development: replacing old blood with new blood plasma, a gene editing procedure called CRISPR, and the whole-body stem cell makeover. But as of 2022, there are major hurdles with each of these. The first two lack extensive human trials and face some controversy for human use and are probably decades away from attaining regulatory approval, and the third, the whole-body stem cell makeover, is prohibitively expensive with a price tag coming in at a whopping $50,000.

The Raw Food Diet

It should be said right up front that the basic raw food diet, 'The Primal Diet' is by itself is a healing diet and it offers life extension benefits. This diet was the diet of our ancestors and the masters of physical immortality, and it is the diet that our bodies are best programmed for. It is a basic raw food diet except for starches and legumes. The Vonderplanitz books, "We Want to Live," and "Recipe for Living Without Disease," give the basics of this raw food Primal Diet, but it consists of raw dairy (unpasteurized milk, cream, cheese, and butter), fresh vegetable juice or daily hearty fresh vegetable salads, fresh fruits, raw (uncooked) eggs, unheated honey, unsalted, unroasted nuts and seeds, and cooked starches and legumes (beans and peas). Life extension diets should avoid all cooked fats, pastries, candy, salt, canned foods and processed foods. At the very least the life extension seeker should make some modifications to their present diet, such as reducing meat consumption or substituting white meat for red meat, reducing cooked fat and processed sugar foods, reducing cooked foods in general, and eating a more wholesome raw food diet.

Lite Water

Lite water, or deuterium depleted water, is a commercial product that has 93% of the heavy water content removed. All waters of world contain approximately 150 parts per million (ppm) of heavy water. Lite water came about when a group of researchers decided to investigate why the Humza people of Pakistan had more centenarians than the other nearby groups. The Humza's themselves said that it was due to their water which was a glacial melt water. When the researchers investigated this, they found that the glacial melt water had 4% less heavy water in it than the worldwide ocean standard which contains approximately 150 ppm of heavy water in it. Studies were done with concentrated heavy water and it was found to be quite toxic. The researchers began to do more studies with lite water and with heavy water and they found in animal studies, when animals were given a water that contained 30% heavy water it immediately caused rapid death. The researchers then tested lite water (with most of the 150 ppm of heavy water removed) on animals and plants and they found that lite water improved the health of the animals and it caused plants to grow larger. Research studies found that heavy water interferes with regeneration. Sources say that the worldwide water standard of 150 ppm of heavy water, is a high amount and it contributes to aging and disease. Lite water with only 10 ppm of heavy water in is commercially available. It not only assists longevity, but it also improves health, and it helps to prevent diseases of all kinds and it has healing properties. It is also said to have an anticancer effect. If the heavy water content can be lowered to only 40 ppm (down from 150 ppm) there are those that say that this will make it difficult for any disease to be able to manifest in the body. Water that has most of the deuterium removed can indeed add years to your life. I have heard that if you drink a water that has been purified to the extent that it contains only 5 ppm of heavy water that this may allow a 200-year life span to open up. An interesting observation that I noticed after drinking 10 ppm lite water for six months was that my damaged toe and finger nails were regenerating once again when before that they were not. When you can bring your body's total heavy water burden down from 150 pm to say 40 ppm, it can markedly assist your body's regeneration and this may help you to reach your natural potential life span of 140 to 150 years. Unfortunately, as of 2022, lite water is expensive.

Radon Health Spas and Mines

Our ancestors as far back as the 12th century were aware of the healing benefits that they experienced when they went down into old abandoned mine shafts that contained trace levels of the slightly radioactive gas radon. Some of these mines in Europe were later developed as radon health mines, and some of the old mining areas were converted into radon health spa resorts, and they have since been operating as healing centers for hundreds of years. Europe has a great many of these radon healing spa resorts and they are accepted for health insurance benefits in many parts of Europe. In the USA, there are several radon health mines in Montana, and Arkansas has a radon hot spring. There are radon hot springs in Canada and there are large number of radon health spas around the world. Literature about the healing properties of radon gas says that the benefit to the tiny capillaries in the body from limited exposure to trace levels of radiation is important and can only be obtained from a series of 1-hour exposures to trace levels of radon gas in the radon health mines or in the radon hot springs. Radon gas and radon embellished water from radon health mines or from radon hot spring spas that contains trace levels of radiation actually stimulates and activates the body's cells, expands the capillaries, improves metabolism, and boosts the body's immunity and natural healing power and these affects are recognized and called radiation hormesis by medical science. Radioactivity carries a rare form of electrical energy deep into the body, bombarding bodily fluids, protoplasm and cell nuclei with energetic explosions of electro-ionized atoms. Cell activity is stimulated and this arouses the secretory and excretory organs and the body expels toxins and waste material. Also, radium in trace levels is a catalyst for destroying some cancer cells and certain toxic bacteria. Radium in the water in trace amounts also benevolently affects the aetheric body and the chakras. It was believed in ancient Atlantis to be so powerful that it was considered to be a life-giving attribute. The Atlanteans believed that what oxygen is to the air, is similar to what radon is to water.

Hyperbaric Chambers, EWOT, and Brown's Gas

In 2020, a study performed in Israel made a worldwide news splash by reporting the anti-aging effects of a clinical trial that involved having test subjects over 60 breathe pure oxygen while being subjected to two atmospheres of pressure (which is 29 psi – pounds per square inch) inside of a hyperbaric chamber. This study became a sensation in media news releases and it proves what has long been known by yoga pranayama breath masters who have utilized breath mastery techniques for extreme longevity. And it is also well known that distance runners maintain a youthfulness far into their maturity. In this Israeli study, 35 people over 64, were given 60 sessions in a hyperbaric chamber over a three-month period. The subjects breathed pure oxygen using face masks while the air pressure in the hyperbaric chamber was maintained at 29 psi. Normal atmospheric pressure is approximately 14.7 psi. This pressurized oxygen saturated their bloodstream and tissues with pure oxygen. The results were not only impressive, but there was an actual age reversal in two aging factors. There was a 20% increase in telomere length and a 37% reduction in senescent cells. The study concluded by saying that the results obtained were similar to the telomere state of a person 25 years younger. This pure oxygen, hyperbaric chamber technology could become a rejuvenation process in the future. An earlier oxygen exercise protocol called EWOT, or Exercise with Oxygen Therapy, also has an anti-aging effect. EWOT exercisers wear a mask that delivers oxygen while they do a work out on an exercise bicycle. Brown's Gas is a gas that consists of two parts hydrogen and one part oxygen and it is obtained by splitting the H2O water molecule using electrolysis. It can be breathed similar to EWOT and there are those who state that it has an even greater anti-aging affect. This is because when H2O water is split apart into its hydrogen and oxygen component gasses, they both briefly exist in the mono-atomic state (H and O) and as such they contain more energy than when they are in their normal bi-atomic state (H-H and O-O). Japan has Brown's Gas spas that list the anti-aging improvements from breathing Brown's Gas, and these include the removal of skin wrinkles and more youthful looking skin and more youthful and healthy-looking body in their clients.

Biochemical Treatments

There is wide range of biochemical treatments and bio-substances available for aging intervention and age reversal. There are literally dozens and dozens of these products on the market and many of them are effective. However, these treatments are expensive and the results are somewhat short lived. Hormone replacement continues to be at the forefront and usually requires medical procedures and treatments. Products such as NAD+ and many, many other bio-chemical substances are available on the internet and other outlets and produce positive results. There may be some contra affects with some of these treatments and a drawback is that they will in the near term continue to be expensive and have short-lived results.

Stem Cell Treatments

Futurists say that the current medical application and knowledge of stem cell treatments is in its infancy. But they also say that when this technology becomes more developed and mature this approach may well be another route to rejuvenation. Interestingly enough, the stem cell method is not limited to only medical science. The ancient masters of immortality were said to be able to release their body's own stem cells for ongoing regeneration to achieve their legendary immortality. Indeed, it is predicted that stem cells will be a major route to rejuvenation for the future human in both the external science and in the internal science after attaining higher consciousness and by using thought-mind-power. Stem cell treatments have now undergone remarkable progress. Stem cells are being used to repair and regenerate damaged or worn-out body parts and are at the beginning stage of growing whole new organs. Dr. Harry Adelson in Utah, USA, offers a 'Full Body Stem Cell Makeover' involving three types of stem cells that are injected all over the body including the spine, scalp, knees, ankles, knees, shoulders, elbows, wrists, hands, etc., and all of this creates a real rejuvenation, and he has a video that clearly shows this process, www.StemCellSolutionFilm.com. Dr. Chan, another stem cell expert adds that organ stem cells are organ specific and to repair and regenerate a specific organ stem cells from that organ must be used.

Gene Editing Interventions

CRISPR/Cas9 is a gene editing technology. It is able to use a guide RNA to locate a sequence in DNA and then use an enzyme called Cas9 to make a cut in the DNA at that sequence location and then either correct the gene or insert a new gene at the cut location. A 2022 Salk Institute report achieved age reversal in middle and older mice using partial cell reprogramming using the Yamanaka factors with no toxicity or adverse side effects. There are four specific genes that encode transcription factors (proteins) called 'Yamanaka Transcription Factors' that can convert somatic cells into pluripotent stem cells that can propagate indefinitely. Transcription factors can turn genes 'on' and 'off' to allow beneficial genes to produce beneficial substances but inhibit genes that produce detrimental substances. A 2022 Yamanaka factors study in human donors around 53 rejuvenated and wound the skin aging clock back about 30 years. And in 2022 research is now underway to rejuvenate older humans using the same technology. The technique is to remove old cells from circulating blood, multiply them and then use transcription factors to transform the old cells back to youthful structure and function, and then reinfuse huge numbers of these reprogrammed stem cells which then induces systemic regeneration. However, there is much controversy from regulatory agencies and the medical community tha questions safety and reliability concerns with this technology, and a few of the early medical researchers have suffered legal penalties.

Removing Old Blood and Adding Young Blood

In a 2005, team of Stanford University researcher found that blood contains more than 50 factors and substances related to aging. They performed a landmark experiment in 2005 in which they surgically connected or cojoined the arteries of a young mouse to the arteries of an old mouse with the astounding result that the old mouse became young again (improved fur color, increased sex drive, better memory, and had the energy of a young mouse), but unfortunately, the opposite occurred to the young mouse – it became pre-maturely old. Indeed, this is a valid approach. But later studies indicated that other factors, such as proximity to the young mouse's organs, may have contributed to the anti-aging results, rather than just the new blood, and when the old mouse only received new blood from the young mouse, the age reversal results were not as good. An interesting and intriguing breakthrough in 2020, was reported by the same Stanford University group that performed the original old mouse, young mouse conjoined arteries study. In 2020, they published a new study showing that some age reversal resulted from simply removing one half of the old blood from the old mouse! This points to the revelation that aging substances and factors exist within old blood. By removing up to one half of this old blood some of the aging it causes can be avoided. Local blood banks in any large city will accept blood donations regardless of age. Anyone can volunteer to be a blood donor and possibly may receive some age reversal benefit. At the present time this approach is being countered by the FDA as unproven, and having no clinical trials. However, many animal studies have been done which report consistent results that demonstrate age reversal when an old animal's old blood is replaced with new young blood or blood plasma from a young animal (and even with human blood plasma). However, there are a number of potential contra indications in any transfusion that warrant caution. As of 2022, clinics offering young blood transfusions from young blood donors have been hindered by the FDA, but research is continuing on this anti-aging approach and will continue.

Body Parts Replacement

Organ and body parts replacement are beginning to be practiced in main stream medicine and they have been a part of sci-fi literature for a very long time, and as we all know sci-fi often transitions into reality. Advanced stem cell work in medical science focuses on organ and body parts repair without the need for surgery. But other methods are also being developed by medical science to regrow lost limbs. The Science Advances journal reported in 2022 that a Wyss Institute science team from Harvard and Tufts Universities were able to regrow a fully functioning frog leg at the leg amputation site in a frog. They put amniotic fluid along with several other growth stimulants in a small cup and attached and sealed this regrowth stimulant solution to the stump in direct contact with the stump tissues for 24 hours period. This triggered regeneration of the frog's leg and after 18 months the frog had regrown a new whole and fully functioning frog leg. Organ and body part replacement is an on-going pursuit in genetic engineering and other sciences and it will become a reality that organs and body parts can be cloned for use in surgical replacement for the sort of immortality that sci-fi writers envision. Many new high-tech technologies for life extension in the future are discussed by futurist. One of them is AI (artificial intelligence) integrated into the brain. This technology may be able to trigger the brain to activate on-going whole-body regeneration for life extension.

Facelift Pens, Water Picks, Cheap Glasses

A google search on plasma pens pulls up a long list of hand-held devices that produce a plasma stream that can remove wrinkles and blemishes. Also, there are ultrasound applicators that can remove skin imperfections and wrinkles through an ultrasonic vibration. There are many wrinkle removing creams on the market that are also affective. Water picks for enhanced dental hygiene have entered the market and are invaluable tools for deep cleansing of the teeth and gums. Cheap plastic glasses have almost become the norm and allow everyone including older people to work on vision demanding computer tasks without having to get expensive glass-based glasses. Hair color products have been available for a century or more and are very effective at transforming gray hair into a vibrant colorful youthful looking hair. There are exercise routines and new exercise devices for increasing bone density for people who suffer from osteoporosis that can increase bone density and reduce the risk of bone fracture. Indeed, it is a wise life extender who takes advantage of these antiaging products and keeps on the lookout for new antiaging arrivals. This is because when you look younger and feel younger it tends to play into your belief system that you actually have become younger.

Healing Sounds, Music, and Color

Sound healing practitioners working with sound frequency formulas can heal and rebalance the body. A two-tone sound formula (two sound frequencies) when played to the body through earphones can rebalance it back into hemostatic. The two-frequency formula approach has also been shown to help heal and regenerate body structures and restore emotional calmness. Sound healing practitioners develop a two-tone sound frequency formula to return an out of balance mental-energy-flow condition back into normal balanced wholeness, and there are predictions that this technology will come into general use. There are also sound healing methods that work with five independent sound frequency vibration combinations and in using this approach it was found that certain five frequency formulas could help repair wounds and damaged or aged body organs, tissues, and structures, and even to some degree regenerate them. Another potential approach using sound involves high amplitude sound vibration that can have a potential rejuvenating affect by disassociating some of the body's cellular structures through the high vibration so that the body can dislodge and remove of some of its old half dead senescence cells that secrete aging substances.

It is well known that beautiful music can bring about a calming and healing and rejuvenating affects though its ability to transmute negative emotional states into calmness, joy and the appreciation of life. And there are visionaries who see a greater use of music and the sounds of nature in hospitals to help set a nurturing tone for healing the body physically and emotionally. It is also well known that bird song and insect sounds have a healing affect and futurist also see the sounds of nature coming to the human population through better urban planning. And they say that these applications with sound will be part of the general longevity and rejuvenation of the future human.

Color is changing into a greater range of colors that display a much greater spectrum of color tints and shades in nature. In the future a flower plant will have beautiful flower blossoms that will spread the basic red or yellow or orange colors into dozens of shades of red or yellow or orange. And this greater spectrum of colors will also be healing and will create a greater joy in experiencing life, and this will also create a desire to live much longer. I have heard futurists say, "Do you know how healing it is to walk through or sit by a beautiful flower garden in full blossom displaying its grand spectrum of tantalizing colors. Indeed!

Crystals, Gold, and a Living Mineral

There are published articles that state that gold and other precious metals were used as part of the complex rejuvenation processes in Atlantis to achieve extremely long-life spans of over 1,000 years. These articles speak about Atlantis Rejuvenation and they say that trace amounts of gold and other precious metals were added to giant 12-foot-high quartz crystals that gave them special properties. One of the applications of these giant crystals was said to be in the rejuvenation process. A crystal, especially one with phi angle facets can greatly help maintain the mental focus needed through thought-mind-power for rejuvenation. Gems are also able to enhance life force energy and thereby enhance longevity. Gems are available to all and they can fortify the aura and balance the chakras. In doing this they can extend life force energy, life potency, and longevity. However, to draw them to you for this use, you must first recognize that the mineral kingdom is alive and sentient in all of its myriad expressions. Within the mineral kingdom there is indeed the spark of divinity, of divine consciousness that is as equally aware in certain aspects as is humanity. This is a fact that is quite true, but is unrecognized by most of mankind.

Phi angle faceted quartz crystals are available and they can enhance your life force energy, fortify your aura, balance your chakras, and help you maintain your mental focus. But in using the phi angle crystals you will need to recognize the consciousness in the crystal and ask it to help you maintain your mental focus in your meditations and in what you desire to manifest. Another item said to be used in Atlantis rejuvenation was a very rare, greenish living mineral substance found only in three places on earth. The largest of these deposits was said to exist as a mineral in deep caverns underneath the Grand Canyon where it was mined and used in the healing and rejuvenation processes of Atlantis. Edgar Casey's readings stated that gems and noble minerals, specifically gold and silver were capable of extending human life. Gold substances can be taken up in the roots of beets and carrots and other long root vegetables and incorporated into their vegetable structures and in this form the gold can be utilized internally in the human body. Since gold is a very good conductor of electricity and energy it is speculated that gold in the vegetable matrix internally in trace amounts in the body may be able to assist in bringing more energy into the body for repair, regeneration and longevity. And wearing gold rings may also assist in bringing in more energy.

The Temple of Rejuvenation

There are articles about the Atlantis Temple of Rejuvenation that say it was a cornerstone rejuvenation processes used during Atlantis. It was said to be combined with other rejuvenation technologies along with higher consciousness and thought-mind-power rejuvenation, and all of this was said to have allowed the Alta-Ra group of Atlantis to attain very long lifespans of over 1,000 years. The Temple of Rejuvenation was as a device that could repolarize the magnetic field of all of the cells of the human body for rejuvenation. It was a large machine and could accommodate six or more people. It was shaped somewhat like a giant football held upright by legs or stilts. Inside and at the center of this giant football was a circular turntable platform that could hold several rejuvenation technicians and their client. Above and below the turntable were large cones which gave the structure its football shape. Wrapped around the cones were many turns of wire or cable that carried a large electric current that produced a powerful magnetic field. The client was strapped to a small massage like table that could be swiveled up and down, and could also rotate around and around. The massage turntable in turn was mounted on the larger main turntable and it was offset from the center of the larger turntable. When the magnetic field was on the client was exposed to the magnetic field and his or her body was rotated by both turntables: the massage table and main turntable. This created a rotation within a rotation inside of a strong magnetic field. The magnetic field permeated the client's body and repolarized and rebalanced the DNA in all of the cells for rejuvenation. During the rejuvenation process, the client's massage turntable would also slowly swivel up and down, from horizontal to vertical and back down again to expose the body to all orientations. This would allow all tissues of the client's body to become repolarized including tissues such as the skin that are responsive to body orientation. This treatment effectively repolarized and rebalanced the client's organs and body for rejuvenation. The rejuvenation was said to last from three to seven years.

Xenon Rejuvenation

There are books that outline the conditions on the earth during the biblical Garden of Eden when mankind did not age and die as it does now. It was said that the main reason for this ongoing perpetuity of the human body was that the Earth's atmospheric reservoir back in those ancient times contained the inert gas xenon at the level of approximately 3% by volume. This xenon gas created a low-level healing and regeneration energy flux that maintained the bodies of the humans in a state of constant healing and regeneration such that there was no aging and death. All of this ended and aging and death begin when the atmosphere no longer contained the xenon gas. Xenon is now one of the rarest gasses in the atmosphere. Few are aware that if xenon gas were reintroduced into the earth's atmosphere at the level of approximately 3% that this healing and regeneration affect would again return, but mankind would still age and die due to the habitual negative thought patterns that mankind harbors and the destructive emotional states that mankind creates. There are a number of techniques to create a xenon energy beam and they involve pressurizing the gas to increase the thermal collisions of the atoms to allow the release of some of the healing xenon energy, and then to subject the pressurized gas to a magnetic field which aligns and directs the energy beam. Indeed, various xenon gas devices will be invented, created and found very useful in healing and regenerating the human bodies of the men and woman of the future.

Rejuvenation with Internal Science

You Can Feel Young and Vital Again

You never cease being. You never end. You are forever ongoing. You can take a deep breath and say, "Well okay, that changes everything. Maybe I can still go surfing or skiing." There is nothing to keep you from being young. You might think that your body gets stiffer with age but you can do yoga exercises to correct that too. Maybe you won't have the same pep that you had when you were younger but that is all in the mind. That is generational teaching and you don't need that anymore. You can act and experience your day as young now as you ever have been. Let that sink in. So, if you want to get up and walk briskly and go for a good workout at a gym and become stronger, go for it. You can feel young again.

As You Evolve You Can Rejuvenate

As you transition into a more evolved man or woman you have the opportunity of rejuvenation. Many of you will get ideas on how to work with the earth and with your dense physical body. They are related. There will be new ideas on how to work with the physical body. You believe rejuvenation to be the reverse of the aging process, but there is more to it than that. It is much more than just reconnecting with your youth or turning back time. It is a harmony with the dense physical body itself, and because the dense physical body is of planet earth, rejuvenation is in harmony with the earth. It is the same type of harmony we are asking you to develop by being conscious of your impact on planet earth. These things are setting you up to take the next step into higher levels of vibration and being. The rejuvenation process is not new to planet earth, and you've done this before. There were many times when you could live to be at least 300 of your years, and if you look at your physical body, it is important to know that it was designed to live that long and longer. It was designed for you to live 300-900 years. So, let us ask, why do you age? A lot of it comes from your belief system which is the actual energy you feed your brain and tell your body it will live this long. Although that seems very simplistic, and it is much deeper than you understand, but changing your belief system is a major key.

Average life spans were once in the 300-year range, and there were even times when humans could actually reach 900 years as mentioned in the Bible! Now people may think that living 900 years is fantastic, but everyone would think nothing of a rock lasting 900 years and the rock is made of the earth too. There are many opportunities for you to start thinking about this in new ways – thinking about moving your body into the new life extension movement. You can start to uncover and work with rejuvenation on different levels. It involves a harmony with the dense physical body itself. You can learn to work with many new ways to bring about an actual rejuvenation for yourself and your human body in the chapters of this book. Also know that it is now more possible than ever before because the earth and humanity have indeed stepped into 5th dimensional awareness even though we are still living in the 3rd dimension. One of the 5th dimensional attributes that you can notice now are the higher vibrational light patterns that you can see in the headlights of cars.

Change Your Thinking to Allow Rejuvenation

We have said it before, but we feel that it is important enough to say it again. When you go about your daily routine: eating, cleaning your teeth, and showering, create thought patterns that your food and drink are nourishing and regenerating for your body, and that the water in your shower is cleansing, healing and rejuvenating every cell in your body. At the breakfast table give thanks for the food you eat and intend that the food will be healthy for you, because the agreement you have that it is healthy for you is more important than what you eat and drink, and also create thought patterns that this food and drink are going to regenerate your body. Put thankfulness in your day every day. Put love and kindness in your day every day. Greet others with a smile and learn to enjoy them. Enjoy driving to work even if there is heavy traffic. Know that anger is like a virus that can infect your body, mind and soul and then go on to infect the world. Then know that love is also like a virus that can infuse your body with it and then infuse the world with peace and joy. On the freeway thought-project peace and patience to all those who cut you off. At work enter with perfect control of your whole system, your mind, body, and soul becoming one with your heart. Feel grateful for your job as you leave work and fill you work area with higher thoughts and emotional patterns. On your way home when you stop for groceries, project loving kindness to the store and all who work there and infuse the food you buy with love and health. Notice that when you do all of these things how it puts you in a framework to allow you to foster your body's ongoing cellular regeneration and rejuvenation. Work on creating this mindset to become a daily habit. Reflect on how creating continual thought streams of healing and rejuvenating showers, and of foods that can nurture and regenerate your body, and of having patience and tolerance while driving to work, and of creating benevolence and goodness at work and shopping, and of giving smiles and feeling enjoyment when interacting with coworkers, family members and others – notice that when you start to do all of this, that it postures you to accept that you can 'youth' and rejuvenate yourself. In doing all of these things, make it a habit to think you are rejuvenating yourself because you can and you are!

You Can Actually Youth Yourself

It is important for you to know this. It is important for you to accept it. It is important for you to surrender to it. And most of all, it is important that you get excited about it! And put a lot of passionate energy into it! That is what will make it work. There is prerequisite for this rejuvenation and it is in keeping your energy intake high. Where does this energy come from? It comes from two main sources: from the food you eat, and from the prana life force energy in the air you breathe in and from the prana that comes in through your chakras if they are open. And your chakras are open when you are happy, feeling creative, being of service and enjoying life. They are partially closed and shut down when you are in conflict about something, worried, depressed, upset or angry. So, to rejuvenate yourself, it is important to keep your chakras open. And working with the six perfections and the nine deep healers can help you to keep them open. Keep your seven chakras open by being happy – allow no drama or trauma. It is important to learn to live with your major and minor chakras fully open. It is also important that you accept the underlying truth that you do have a higher dimensional spirit body that is apart from and separate from the aging process. Aging is a lower 3rd dimensional process. Your spirit body is higher dimensional and it does not grow old, it never grows old. It is also important that you surrender your old beliefs that aging is mandatory. It is not. There are many ways to keep your body in the state of middle age maturity almost indefinitely. Your beliefs form your thought patterns which create your reality. Can you rejuvenate? Of course, you can, but you must maintain beliefs that it is possible, and that you deserve it. And after that you must create the expectancy that you are going to do it. There is a certain cockiness to this also. And you must surrender the old paradigm of tending see the world as malevolent and full of dangers and hazards. You must begin to open up and see the evolving world as beneficial and helpful and benevolent and beautiful – it is a beautiful blue jewel as seen from space.

Choose to Rejuvenate Just One Cell of Your Body

When you choose to recreate and rejuvenate just one cell of your body, it is much easier on your belief system then to try to rejuvenate your entire body all at once. Your belief system can probably accept this and say, "Well, okay, I could probably mentally picture just one of my cells and mentally see it rejuvenated." And then it is just another step to allow that one rejuvenated cell to become a master template that can instruct all of your other body cells to do the same. This is much easier on your belief system. You can also choose to visualize just one stem cell inside of that cell being activated and becoming a brand-new cell.

You Must Be Passionate About It

You must allow a slight smile to grace your face as you come to realize that indeed this is going to make a real difference and keep you in an on-going state of mature youthfulness. You must really relish the idea of keeping yourself passionately youthful. Can you do this? Can you get passionate about it?

You Must Be Consistent with It

Once you have the basis of this inner science rejuvenation technique you must be consistent and impeccable with it. You must start a new cycle of yourself. You can't one day think, "This is great, I am rejuvenating myself," and then the very next day think, "Who am I kidding?" You must keep the frequency. You can't go back and forth like that and expect it to work. It will work when you are able to be impeccable about keeping the frequency. It is very good to build up a powerful unshakable knowledge base of your past successes in always being able to create what you want to manifest by using the power of your mind. You can start by manifesting simple things such as, say manifesting say, a purple circle. You can say, "I intend to manifest a purple circle," and then watch how it manifests. Your spirit guides may impulse you to notice a purple circle in an advertisement, or on the cover of a magazine, or a discarded paper in a playground, or send you an impulse to shop at a store where you can find some. That is the play of it— that is the beginning of thought-manifestation. In advanced thought-manifestation practices, you can actually create material things out of the aethers. So, you can certainly manifest rejuvenating just one cell. And then you simply tell that one cell to go and tell all of the others to do the same thing and rejuvenate. The best way to youth and rejuvenate is on a schedule that you choose and you should plan on doing it say, one day a week for a month. And then after that, you should do it periodically, say once or twice a year. I suggest that when you do the youthing visualization-meditation below, follow it up by saying the rejuvenation affirmation that follows out loud in low voice. Perhaps choose a certain time that you will do them. And then, the night before you do your youthing meditation and rejuvenation affirmations, you might think about it and build up your excitement and passion for it.

Youthing Meditation

Goggle human cells so you have an image of what one of them looks like and can visualize it. Stare at it for several minutes to add beginning concentration. Assume your meditative posture, slow your breathing, invite your spirit team to help, and become as still as you can—become as still as a statue if possible. Go deep into your body and visualize just one cell and the DNA inside that cell. Now, very firmly and with the command of a general, speak the words below loud enough so that you and your primal energy field and your body cells and your whole body can all hear it. Say to that one cell, "Beautiful cell of mine, we are going to go on a new program. I instruct you to youth—to rejuvenate back to your youthful template." Hold that image for a while, as long as you can. Your cells are all connected. That one cell will communicate your instructions to all the other cells. Now put a smile on your face, and with a certain cockiness in your personality, come out of the meditation and allow an expectation that it is starting to happen and that is all there is to it!

Next, you should bolster your rejuvenation meditation with the rhyming rejuvenation affirmation below. Some of the words in it are important. The word 'accept' means that you accept a condition and are not in denial of it. You need to accept that you have an ageless light body that never grows old, and you do. The word 'surrender' means you will let go of your resistance to this and your old limiting beliefs. It is important to lean into the notion of surrendering the old pattern of aging. The word 'choose' is linked to your first chakra, your root chakra, your foundation. When you choose to do something, it becomes your new foundation. It becomes that which you have chosen to become. Do you follow? When you use the word 'choose' you are in the process of creating whatever it is that you want to create. The words, 'I can' are the vibration and energy of excitement. Whenever you say the phrase 'I can', it connotes the meaning of something that you want to do or want to accomplish is within your abilities. When used in the rhyming affirmation below it suggests that this is something that you can do. When you do this for a long time you create a new cycle of yourself, and this creates a new belief system, a new mental self-image of you, a new thought projection cycle of you...and all of this will rejuvenate you!

Youthing Rhyming Affirmation
I accept that I have a light body that never will grow old.
I surrender old beliefs that we all must age as I was told.
I choose to recreate and youth and rejuvenate my body now!
I absolutely can youth and I positively don't need to know how!

This will work because you are the boss of your body. You can tell it what you want it to do, and it will follow your instructions. Your belief system is a key to all of this. And so, to help your belief system accept that it is possible, you should also do as many of the other things in this book that you that you know will help your longevity, such as converting to a better diet that fosters better cell regeneration (your personal variation of the raw food diet), your own fasting program, your own breathwork practices, keeping yourself reasonably physically fit, incorporating a longevity lifestyle, getting rid of your death urge, and enjoying life to the fullest. You should also do the visualization exercises, and mediations, and instruction sets in this book that you that you know are going to help your longevity. When you do all of these things it will help your belief system immensely to believe that it is indeed possible for you to also youth yourself. These things all work together you know. You should do them enough so that it cognates and becomes you.

After you do your initial youthing meditation and affirmation, I suggest that you do a follow up youthing meditation and affirmation periodically, at least once a year, better is twice a year. Give it a try! You won't be sorry. Do the meditation, and then say the rhyming affirmation 3 or 4 times each times each time you work with this. After a year goes by you should be pleased with your progress, particularly if you add many of the other things for longevity that go alone with it that you have read about in this book and in other articles, books, and other sources. Next add playfulness. Be playful, have fun. Do the things you really enjoy doing. Bring in things that remind you of when you were in your youth, such as high school or college clothes, songs from your youthful years. Really get into it. Act like you would act if you were younger. Add laughter. Add humor. Find things to laugh about. Add socializing. Don't worry about how old you are. Incorporate the playfulness a young person has. Get involved with life again as though you were a more youthful person again. Make plans for the future that you want to make since you are youthing!

Now add circle energy. Expand into your new belief system. Remember you have to change your old patterns and your old belief system and your old expectation, and you need to have a zest for life. You need to expand into your new zest for life. You are hereby given a second chance to live outside the box of your culture's limiting beliefs about how long you can live. You have to agree to change your concepts about life and what it means to you to stay alive in a youthful mature body for a long, long, long time. The youthing meditation and the rhyming youthing affirmation, will allow more life-force energy to flow into your body through your chakra system and this will affect the vibration of every cell in your body. With this extra energy in your body, you truly do have a magic wand. Let this wand recreate the youth that you want. And so let it be.

The life extension seeker should also be open to trying some of the new external technologies that have become available. There will be more discoveries and inventions coming along to help men and women live longer. The serious life extension student should do the youthing meditation and affirmation exercise periodically and keep it in their anti-aging toolbox as an important on-going life extension practice.

CHAPTER 11

It Is Possible to Live Over 500 Years

Masters say it's possible to live over 500 of your years.
Some of you were trained in this – eons upon eons ago.
You will need to mimic the masters and forget your peers.
You will need to practice what the masters taught eons ago,
But most won't follow the masters due to social censure fears.
But you can work with new life extension revelations and know
That they can assist you to slow your aging even if old age nears
Or, you can opt for rejuvenation technologies that will soon show,
And triple your life span (such is the claim for them) – as it appears.
Or you can go for the gold and emulate the immortal masters of old
Who mastered the mind and the breath and the long fast we are told
And reached life spans that seemed a sort of immortality of over 500 years
Which so astounded the masses that they were immortalized by their peers.
But, think of it! Think of being able to reach a 500-year life span!
You would surely be a way shower by demonstrating that you can!

Immortality – A New Beginning and a New Awakening

As mankind awakens to higher consciousness and learns about the power of love to heal the body and keep the body healed, and as people hear more about humans beginning a cycle of longer lives, these ideas of life extension and physical immortality will soon become more attractive than the old death and reincarnation cycle. For many older people, the idea of life extension will have more to do with the fear of their own impending death, but for others, the realization that the current life spans are just far too short to get done what they need to do will be the reason. We can ask if the dawning of the Age of Aquarius is going to be the springboard for humans to actually heal deeply enough to heal into physical emotional and mental perfection such that they will be able to move into life extension and a sort of physical immortality? By healing, it is meant that profound and deep, deep healing is one of main themes and goals for this new age, and it is a prerequisite for life extension and for physical immortality. This deep, deep healing is broad based and pervasive and it includes healing the planet and all of the life forms that live upon her also, not just mankind. While most humans have not awakened anyway near their inborn capacity to heal and rejuvenate themselves, they are slowly beginning to hear this and they will eventually come to know this truth. And indeed, every day people are healing themselves from potentially lethal disease conditions. From a spiritual perspective healing is simply the act of purifying the physical, emotional and mental bodies from the diseased states that they previously experienced. In every physical healing, some complementary healing must also take place in the consciousness as well, since consciousness with its emotional and mental bodies is most often the root cause in the first place, and the entire consciousness must also enter into wholeness as well in order to support the physical healing

Perfecting the Physical, Emotional, and Mental

Physical and emotional perfection, and the perfection of the mentality are states whereby the physical body and the emotional, mental consciousness that inhabits it, have been thoroughly purified of all disease and all aging and all of the death impulses such that the body is allowed to reach a state of immortality whereby the body does not age and die, but instead is allowed to continue on and on and on. But aging and death are the pervasive and the accepted experiences. Even after humans realize that immortality can be a possibility, it usually takes another three to four lifetimes to completely purify the body and the mind of the death imprint. But starting now is the best approach. Beyond what most people think is possible is an immense and unimaginable field of unrealized possibilities and potentials. And in nearly every spiritual tradition that has come to the earth there have been masters and adepts who did bring their physical bodies to perfection. And there are scriptures (Hebrew, Ecclesiastes, Ecc 3:11) that state," God hath put eternity into the heart of man." Humanity has always sought to learn and attain the ability to have a deathless continuation. One of the earliest known texts ever recorded, the Sumerian "Epic of Gilgamesh," is about hero's journey to search for his immortality. Indeed, the quest to attain immortality has continued down through the long ages of the human race and in modern times it is being pursued in earnest by medical science. Why doesn't this ever fall out of fashion? Why hasn't humanity just given up on it?

Sri Aurobindo and the Mother's Spiritual Light

Sri Aurobindo realized that immortality could be attained by a human who had worked with and mastered all of the five stages of his ladder of ascending consciousness and he saw that if the seeker was able to fully attain the fifth level (total integration of body-mind-emotion-spirit) he or she could attain physical immortality. His spiritual partner who he called 'The Mother' held that achieving physical immortality was her life mission, and much of her own inner work centered around daily filling her physical body or vessel with light. As time went on, although she did not attain physical immortality, she did succeed in filling her physical vessel with great amounts of spiritual light that she so diligently drew to herself and accumulated that it became a physical reality for her so much so that it could actually be seen and felt by those who attended her. And certainly, accumulating spiritual light, or prana life force energy, is a complimentary aspect of attaining physical immortality.

Historical Examples of Perfection

Historically, the idea of physical immortality has seen many emotional reactions that range somewhere between utter disbelief and suspicion to outright rage. However, the human beliefs about how long a person can live are now beginning to change, and slowly but surely people all over the world are beginning to find the idea of bodily perfection linked to life extension intriguing rather than impossible, and indeed, there have been those who have demonstrate it.

There have been those who were called immortals who have appeared in the literature from time to time. It is said that students of the great teacher in both Atlantis and Egypt, Thoth, maintain that he was able to keep the same body for over a thousand years, but today this considered legend. Another famous case is that of Babaji of India who manifested a body for himself in India in 1970. He taught purification practices to his disciples with the goal of reaching physical immortality. Babaji could materialize and dematerialize his body at will and he would appear to his students no matter where they were. Although he lived in India, he also appeared to a few Western students such as Leonard Orr on a few occasions. It is also true that there were some Western saints who were able to bilocate and even tri-locate. This ability is a form of body perfection, because it demonstrates mastery over matter and space. Another is St Germaine who is an ascended master and who from time to time manifested a physical body for a mission on Earth, and he has confounded historians due to his appearances being recorded over a 250-year period.

The idea of body perfection or physical immortality typically will trigger a sense of an impossible goal for most because disease and death have been the reality and way of it for almost all of humanity's history from 30,000 years ago to present. But people today are being worked with to create the model of the future human, those who will walk upon the future awakened Earth, and it is time now to rise to the occasion and release the deep-seated notion that death is an unescapable reality, and it can be discovered that at all levels in the journey to a perfected body, that it requires less effort and more joy than the old way of simply aging and dying.

Musing on Living a Thousand Years

This is a time now of being ignited by higher energies moving through your physical bodies, and this is not your energetic body, it is your physical body—your physicality. You are indeed multidimensional, but you have this body that encases you and you came here to enjoy it—to fully experience all that can enjoyed through your senses of touch, taste, smell, sound, and hearing. You are here not just to know pain, but you are here to also know the ecstatic state of physical reality, of how good your skin feels, of how beautiful are the sights and smells of flowers, of how wonderful the majestic sounds of an orchestra sound, of how delicious some foods, meals, and recipes can taste, and of course the ecstasy, ecstasy, ecstasy of your sexual unions. When you fully understand that being physical is a precious gift, the most precious gift you have, then you may indeed come to want to live far longer than the current culture is programmed for—even far past life extension, up far, far longer—even say, to possibly a thousand years! Yes, and it will eventually become possible for you to eventually actually learn how to live for a thousand years through many avenues: mastering the inner science of physical immortality, utilizing the coming rejuvenation technologies, and working with the powerful antiaging revelations presented in this book and others! Did you hear that? You can learn to live in your physical body for a thousand years once you fully accept your body as a precious gift. Your multidimensional being says 'yes' to the third dimension, but it also says 'yes' to the 4th, 5th and 6th and all of the higher dimensions. It does not say I only want to experience the third dimension. It says I want to experience it all, and I am grateful for all.

The 3rd dimension has such a high death urge—so much so that most people want to leave it—but you forget that this is the dimension of your physical yumminess. Yes, it is but most of you doubt how beautiful and delicious it can be. Most of you tend to say, "Let me leave it." But as a life extender, you must stop wanting to leave. Indeed, you must learn to cultivate the beauty and deliciousness of your sojourn here on Earth. You must start to say, "Let me stay and experience more, and more, and more. Let me taste, and feel, and hear, and touch, and sense more. Let me experience in physicality all the benefits of being physical."

It is also very important to fully fathom that your body is always healthy. Health is your natural, normal state. It is your beliefs about your body that cause it to be not healthy. Your body is always whole as its natural state as you are in the 3rd dimension, and also in the 4th, 5th and higher dimensions. You are always whole. It is your beliefs and your negative emotions and negative thought patterns that cause you to move out of wholeness. Your responsibility is to remember that your body is a gift and not something to let go of. Living for a thousand years in a physical body that is healthy when you have learned how to benefit from all of the things physical, is magic! This is magic: each touch, every smell, all that you taste, and all that you hear. These are your senses. This is your sensuality. This is your deliciousness. To Live a Thousand Years—**Honor your Body**.

Your body can be just as perfect now in the physical as it can be in the spiritual and in the higher dimensional realms. Your body contains a lightbody. Hear this deeply: your body contains a lightbody, and in the higher dimensions everyone wears lightbodies. Honor your body and experience its beauty. That which you are looking for you already have. Do you want to have the highest experiences or perform miracles or have peace in your daily life? You can do all of that now, but you must not say, "I wish to go to heaven." You must say, "This is heaven. I am an angel now on Earth, and I do not need to leave my physical body to become something else, because I am all of it now. I have a physical body to experience the dimensional curiosity, to experience what it is like to see and feel and touch and hear."

It is very good to say, "I am going to drink a glass of water, and I will feel it within my body. My cells will expand from the water, and I will feel it. I sense that this water came from the Earth and the clouds. The water is part of the Earth's process and I am one with this experience." Or you might eat a salad and know that someone planted a seed and a plant grew from it, and now you are deliciously tasting this gift and your body experiences and relishes it. Or you might hear beautiful music and begin to think about the composer who created it and revel in the gift that music offers in that it expresses some of the feelings and experiences of the one who created it. It is important to know that all of these things, and many, many others, are of great beauty and to relish this beauty. This is what you are honored to experience in the 3rd dimension and this is the reason why you might want to choose to live a thousand years. And growing into an ongoing appreciation of what has been created before in all of the many areas of expression and then diving into what is now being created, written, invented, developed and brought into the world is exciting. It is highly exciting! When you truly desire to be a part of it, you can be a part of it. And when you can see that it makes you happy and playful and joyful to work with and become a part of the new world, the new creation, you will want to live longer perhaps even to a thousand years. And indeed, in this book there are so many practices and processes that you can learn and use to extend your life with, and you are now beginning to take baby steps towards doing it. And when you combine those processes with the joy in your heart that you want to live much, much longer, that is what, indeed, will begin to make it possible and happen.

You can live a thousand years in your physical body once you begin to say, "I am physical and I am happy to be physical. I am also happy to have higher dimensions all the way up to the 12th working with me." Now occasionally you may have an experience that is not too good for you in some way, but you can look at it as a new experience, as something different and then move on. You can know that there is much, much more to experience, and it is not as important as it may seem at the time. Allow yourself to understand that if you live in your physical body for a thousand years, any negative thing that happens in the next few months or next few years means very little. Honor yourself and honor others for choosing to be here. Honor yourself for agreeing to be physical at a time when it is not a positive thing to be physical. It is a time when most people say, "I wish to go to heaven, or I wish to be taken up in a ship, or I wish I could be out of this body." You choose to experience time when it only seemed that humans could live 70, 80, 90 or possibly a hundred years. But living to a thousand years is a truth, a real possibility, if you honor your physical body as a lightbody and if you cultivate the enjoyment of allowing all of your senses: sight, hearing, smell, touch, taste (and believe it or not, more are coming!) to have their full expression and if you honor your physical body as a lightbody, because in truth it really is.

Advanced Life Extension with Thought-Mind-Power

There Is the Potential to Become Nearly Immortal

There really is. And it will involve advanced immortality practices using thought-mind-power. Literature exists that alludes to the very long-lived sect in Atlantis called the Alta-Ra, and in addition to their Temples of Rejuvenation they also used thought-mind-power rejuvenation. And they used phi-cut crystals to help them maintain the necessary concentration with this. In Atlantis, it was said that trace amounts of gold and other precious metals were added to the giant 12-foot-high quartz crystals that gave special properties to the crystals, and some of them were said to be another part of the complex rejuvenation process that was used in Atlantis to help them achieve life spans of over a thousand years.

Phi-cut crystals are available now in our time. Crystals, especially those with phi-cut angled facets, can help you maintain the mental focus needed for this though-mind-power rejuvenation. It might be a wise investment to obtain one of them for this advanced rejuvenation with the thought-mind-power process. High consciousness and a highly developed mental focus were said to be important aspects and abilities of the extremely long-lived Alta-Ra sect of Atlantis, and they were needed for the thought-mind-power rejuvenation process that was perfected in Atlantis. The technique for creating rejuvenation through thought-mind-power is to develop prefect knowledge of what the organs of your body look like, how they are constructed, how they should function, and how they should interface and work with the other body systems that they are connected to. There are now many good anatomy books that can help you begin to develop this perfect knowledge of your body's anatomy and what it should look like, and how all of its parts should go together, and how each of its parts should function. You will need to obtain good human body anatomy books with many pictures and illustrations in them and then you can start to try to master the rejuvenation of your organs and body through the thought-mind-power process. You will first need to study the illustrations and memorize them to some degree. You will need to memorize what your major organs look like and know how they should function.

The technique is to begin to use your imaging ability to image (to imagine) one of your organs in the detail shown in the anatomy book illustrations and then superimpose that image over your own organ. You will in a sense recrystallize your organ into its more perfected design. And then you will need to speak in a low voice to your primal energy field, and to your whole body as an entity, and to that particular organ, and to all of the cells in it, and to all of the connections to it; and then state that we as a 'we-ness' whole are going to recreate that organ and bring it back to designed perfection. You should do this one organ at a time in the beginning. Later, when you have developed mastery at this you can do more and even all of your whole body.

We will also add to this a meditation technique in which you totally dissolve your existing body into a blue-light cocoon. This is a very powerful healing tool that can be very useful to heal any condition whatsoever that needs healing, even aging. Indeed, and the underlying visualization of an electro-magna-aetheric blue-light cocoon is connected to the primal blue light life force energy that envelopes and sustains all life forms on Earth and can be seen as a blue aura from space.

If you can obtain a phi-cut crystal, it would be very helpful to add it to this meditation. If you have one you will need to program it for this rejuvenation. Work with your crystal by acknowledging the consciousness that indwells in it and ask it to help you maintain your mental focus. You may be surprised to find that you ability to concentrate is indeed improved when using it.

Thought-Mind-Power Blue Cocoon Rejuvenation

Obtain an anatomy book, decide which organ in your body you want to rejuvenate and gaze at the illustrations of it for several minutes memorizing to the best of your ability all of the details of it and all of its connections to the other parts of your body, and cognate how it should function in its perfected state. Go to your sacred place, assume your meditation position, calm yourself to stillness, slow your breathing, hold your phi-cut crystal if you have one, and bring in your spirit team. Visualize that you are surrounded by blue light energy and become totally and completely enveloped in a cocoon of electro-magna-aetheric blue light that saturates every organ, every, tissue, every cell, every molecule, every atom, and the spaces between the atoms. Now, focus on and visualize the organ you want to rejuvenate being enveloped and slowly dissolving into this blue light energy. This cocoon of blue light totally permeates and saturates you and the organ you are rejuvenating, and it extends six inches outside of your skin in all directions. This blue light is very, very strong and your body and the organ slowly begins to dissolve and dematerialize into it. See your body dissolve. See that organ dissolve. They dissolve, dissolve, dissolve into this blue light until only the nonphysical template is left. When your body has completely dissolved into this cocoon of blue light, the template shadow form of your body pulses with each breath… pulses, pulses, pulses.

Now focus on that organ or body part that you want the bring back into perfection and rejuvenation and use your thought-mind-power concentration abilities to superimpose your perfected image of that organ (from the anatomy book) over the dissolved template of it. Hold this superimposed visualization as long as you can.

And then allow that organ and your body to slowly, slowly, slowly begins to recrystallize with the intent that it recrystallizes back into its perfected form from its master template and your memory of the anatomy book organ – totally healed, totally whole, and without any aging degeneration. Slowly, slowly, slowly recrystallize it and your whole body back into its perfected form, in perfect alignment, in perfect balance, in its perfected system of organs and tissues and structures to work as a whole, integrated, healed and rejuvenated physical body part. Slowly come back with your superimposed perfected image of that organ and intend that this transmutation begin.

This is advanced use of the power of Universal Law of Thought. This is fully understanding that the Universal Law of Thought is the creative essence of all things. Thought is that which creates. It is the creative force of the universe.

Edgar Cayce predicted more than seven decades ago that humans would begin to evolve into a new physical format, a new body type after 1998, and this is happening right now. And after 2038 it will make another leap into another higher body format. The closer you come to the 2038 crossroads, the greater the vibrational, gravitational and dimensional change will be. We as a race of humans on the earth are a young race and as we evolve into a more mature race, and become more integrated into a more benevolent civilization, we will as Cayce predicted, be able to live much, much longer and life extension will apply to the majority of the world's population.

Secrets of the Immortal Masters - The Long Fast

The Long Fast – a key to Immortality

I have heard it said many times that for some of you it will be very important to become way showers for the new life extension that is coming to the planet. This new life extension or an immortality of sorts will come from several different directions. Some will attain it through mastering the immortality practices of the ancient masters. Others will reach it with the new rejuvenation technologies that are being developed. Some will youth through mastery of the recently revealed interdimensional wisdom. And there will be others who will rejuvenate themselves from their own stem cells when they reach the consciousness level such that their DNA works at 88%.

And there will be a few who will reach it by using one of the secrets of the ancient immortal masters, and one of the major techniques of the master was the long fast. Leonard Orr's book, "Physical Immortality," was my introduction to one of the practices that the masters in India used to attain extreme longevity or a near immortality. A master named Babaji, taught Leonard purification practices including fasting. Leonard went to India to work with Babaji and learn physical immortality from him. At the end of Leonard's first trip to India, Babaji told Leonard that he must fast one day a week for one whole year. Leonard picked Monday because he had fewer social obligations on Monday. Monday is also my choice. Leonard fasted every Monday for a whole year. And then he went back to India to see and work with Babaji a second time and learn more. At the end of Leonard's second trip, Babaji told Leonard, "Now you must fast three days a week for a whole year." Leonard wrote that he broke down at the halfway point, but recovered and finished the year. I was resolved and stalwart and I did not break down. I fasted three days a week for a whole year.

But that was all I learned about fasting from Leonard and Babaji. Years later, I read another book, "The Wandering

Taoist," which was about a Taoist community that lived on top of a high plateau in China. This book had a chapter on meeting the immortals. One day, the author, (who at the time was a young Taoist acolyte) was taken to meet the immortals by the Grand Master. As a way of introducing them, the Grand Master said, "Some of them can fast for three months, consuming nothing but water and herbal tea." More years went by before I came upon Herbert Shelton's books on fasting, especially his, "Fast and Grow Young." In it, Shelton relates a study performed on a group of worms in which the life span of two groups of worms were monitored and compared. The first group was allowed to continually feed, but the second group was alternately fed--fasted, fed--fasted, fed--fasted throughout the study. The results were astonishing! The fed-fasted group outlived the continually fed controls by seventeen times! Did you hear that, the fed-fasted group outlived the continually fed group **seventeen times**!

Shelton then related his own experiences as a fasting supervisor at the Hygienic Clinics. He witnessed the rejuvenation benefits he always observed in his clients who underwent a long fast. As part of his duties as a fasting supervisor, he supervised many fasts of 40 days, 50 days, and even a few that went 60 days. And he always noticed that not only did his client's health improve, but he also noticed the rejuvenation affects that always accompanied their long fast. His books vividly describe the rejuvenation he witnessed in his clients after they underwent a fast of over 40 days. There was always a rejuvenation affect. He observed that his client's eyesight improved, their sexual function was restored, their cardiovascular measurements were better, and there were many other health and healing benefits observed and measured.

Shelton explained that the body has two systems for supplying nutrients to its vital organs. The first is, of course, digestion. But the second (not so well known) is a ketone process that breaks down fat reserves and recycles the nutrients in them to feed the vital organs: the heart, lungs, kidneys, liver, and the brain. And as the fast continues, the ketone process breaks down other non-vital tissues to recycle the nutrients in them to feed the vital organs so that the vital organs are always fed. Medical science is also beginning to realize that when old senescent cells are removed from the body, the aging secretions that they release is stopped. And when fasting experts such as Shelton witnessed rejuvenation in his clients who underwent long fasts of 40, 50, 60 days, what happened was that some of the old senescent cells were eliminated, and the toxic substances that they create were removed. Also, with some of the old senescent cells gone, the space that they occupied becomes available for new cells.

The old saying that what can be done with external science can also be done with internal science is real. The immortal masters in ancient times had no technology. And yet there are legends of them living 500 to 900 years. Many people have a hard time believing this, but when you begin to read books on fasting – especially the long fast, what you start to realize is that it is indeed possible!

My 1st Long Fast, 4-Weeks or 28-Days

In January 2019, I decided to do the shortest of what I term the long fast, and so I chose to do a 4-week fast. And right after I had completed it, it was revealed to me in a dream from the higher dimensions that my long fast was the way to go for it, if I wanted to go for a great leap in life extension. The my dream, a kind and firm voice said very plainly, "Why not go for it? Why not go for more than 200 years? Why not go for it and go for 300 years?!"

This was, I believe, a revelation from a higher dimensional master to let me know that I was on the right track, and that if I wanted to live that long (300 years) the long fast was the way to go for it. My first 4-week long fast was hard, especially the fourth week. I seemed to have no energy. But, surprisingly enough, at the beginning of my 4-week long fast, after the fourth day, I was never hungry. In fact, I was never hungry after the fourth day all throughout the remaining weeks! After the fourth day the body begins to feed its vital organs from the ketone break down process with the nutrients that can be recycled from the fat reserves and later from the non-vital tissues. But, I found that the 4th week was the hardest. When I got near the end of the fast, I found myself anxious to start eating again. And then I found that breaking a long fast is not an easy thing to do. As soon as I had completed the 4th week, I wanted to eat way too much and that can be dangerous. It is important to break a long fast as slowly as you can and this does take will power.

My 2nd Long Fast, 5-Weeks or 35-days

In January and February of 2020, I did my second long fast. My second long fast of 5-weeks or 35 days went better than I expected. Again, I was not hungry after the 4th day. I should say though that after the first two weeks, it becomes a little difficult to speak because your mouth gets dry. This is a little awkward at first but you get used to it. I found that having a water bottle nearby to wet my mouth helped. Again, the last week, the 5th week, was the hardest. I felt weak and had low energy. I looked forward to the day when it was over. Again, I found it hard to limit the amount of food I wanted to eat the day I broke the fast. And this time I noticed that the 4th week was not so bad after all. It was about the same as the 3rd week, and the 2nd week. And this time I kept my fast to myself and told very few about it, especially fellow employees and coworkers at my workplace.

My 3rd Long Fast, 6-Weeks or 42-days

In January and February of 2021, I did my third long fast. Prior to starting it, I confided to a coworker that I had done a 4-week long fast in 2019, and a 5-week long fast in 2020. After hearing this she inquisitively asked, "Are you going to do a 6-week fast this year?" And so, after thinking about that, I thought, "Why not? Why not go for it? Why not go for a 6-week long fast this time and break my previous year's record?" And so, I did. And it went better! After the two previous long fasts, I was steeled in my resolve to eat no food whatsoever for the duration of my 6-week long fast. However, there are those who say that you can have a small amount of juice, and I tried that, and I found that it tends to undermine and interfere with the goal of the long fast which is to allow the ketone process to break down as much non-vital tissue as possible. I did drink a lot of lite water and I think this adds even more to the cleansing of the long fast. This time I was able to expect that I would have enough energy from the daily break down products to get through each day of the week at work and that is exactly what happened and it just became a daily routine. There will be always be a problem with speaking during your long fast because your mouth gets dry, but you can still talk with a little effort, and having a water bottle nearby helps. And again, the last week was the hardest, but all of the prior weeks were not so bad. And again, I was anxious to start eating again, but this time after breaking the fast I had a little more control and it went better.

My 4th Long Fast, 7-Weeks or 49-days

In January and February of 2022, I did my fourth long fast and this one went 49 days. I found to my surprise that my body had begun to adapt to it. It became more routine. I told no one at my workplace. But I began to tell others outside my workplace that: "Now I am in my 20s," meaning in day 20 through day 29… and so on up to, "now I am in my 40's," meaning day 40 through day 49. Again the 7th week was the hardest and the earlier weeks that were so hard in previous years were not so hard this time. And again, it was still an effort to limit the amount of food and drink that I wanted to consume after the fast was over. But the results were better, a deeper cleansing was noticed, and greater tear down of old tissues was accomplished.

Comments About My Long Fasts

I find that it always takes my body several weeks to fully readjust to eating again. Most literature on fasting, especially fasting for over a month recommends having a doctor monitor your progress to make sure that fasting is not causing you any harm. I do not feel this is necessary for a number of reasons. The main reason is that if you work up to the long fast slowly you will know how you are doing. The concern I have about having a doctor monitor your fast is that you will be subjected to the belief system of the medical establishment with all of its limitations. I also do not recommend talking about doing a long fast (or a short fast either) to anyone at your workplace for the same reason. I suggest just doing it, and not bragging about it, and not even talking about it. It tends to frighten people and they will try to talk you out of it. You want to do the fast to reap the anti-aging benefits you can get from it and you don't want to get talked out of it. And if you do bring it up in casual conversation you are sure to invite that. What I do suggest is that you work up to it slowly. I suggest that you start with the 1-day a week fast. Masters who teach physical immortality say that the 1-day a week fast should become a lifelong habit. It is for me. I fast 1-day a week every week and I have been doing this for 25 years now. But I am not a fanatic about it either. I don't fast during vacations or holidays. But, outside of that, most every Monday will find me fasting approximately 32 hours.

How Do You Start Fasting?

I would suggest that fasting beginners start with the 1-day a week fast. However, many find this too hard to do, and Intermittent Fasting, which has become quite popular in recent years may be another avenue that you can use to get started in fasting. When you are beginning your fasting practice, I suggest doing the 1-day a week fast for at least three months. And then after that when you get used to the 1-day a week fast and it becomes routine, you can increase it to a 3-days a week fast for several months. Yes, 3-days a week, every week for a month or two. You will find that you can tough it out. Then revert back to the 1-day a week fast for a few months. After you've accomplished that, you can go for a longer fast, perhaps a week-long, 7-day fast. You will find that you can actually survive that. After you accomplish a 7-day fast, revert back to the 1-day a week fast for another month or so. And then after you prove to yourself that you can do it and get used to the 1-day a week fast, and that you can tough it out through a 3-days a week fast, and that you can even survive a 1-week fast; then perhaps you will be ready to go for a longer fast. At first, go for a 2-week fast. And then go for a 4-week fast like I did. Gradually you will find that it's all doable. Doing the 1-day a week fast always, and periodically doing the long-fast is a secret of the ancient immortal masters!

How Does the Long Fast Rejuvenate the Body?

The long fast requires your body to scavenge upon itself to supply recycled nutrients to the vital organs. After the body's fat reserves are used up, the long fast disassembles and breaks down the tissues and substances in the cells of the non-vital tissues including the old senescence cells and it uses whatever nutrients it can from the breakdown products to feed the vital organs: the heart, lungs, liver, kidneys, brain, etc. And in doing this it purifies the blood. And, as we have said, in scavenging on the body's non-vital tissues, it also disassembles and removes some of the old half dead senescence cells that secrete a cascade of aging substances, and it does all of this naturally. This break-down process also removes deeply buried toxins from the physical body. In addition, any overweight burden is reduced or eliminated. All of these benefits add up to better health and increased longevity. Shelton's books on fasting document many health issues (well over 60) that are cured and healed during the long fast. Indeed, many health problems are reversed, including all types of heart disease, diabetes, hearing and vision problems, sexual dysfunction, arthritis, and many, many others. The long fast is one of the secrets of purification and mastery of the physical, mental and emotional bodies for purification and life extension. It demonstrates mastery of the mind over body. And after all it does take quite a bit a mastery to be able to will yourself to do all of this. And as I have already stated, all of you reading this have the potential and ability to become masters.

How Long Can a Human Live Without Food?

Current medical articles say about 90 days, or about three months. But if you incorporate pranayama breathing techniques into your fasting, I would speculate that it should be possible to go longer. It is important to know that the greater portion of the energy that fuels your body does not come from food. In fact, the masters say that the majority of the energy that fuels your body comes in from the prana or life force energy that you breathe in with your breath and the prana that comes in through your open chakras. So, if you do some of the breathing practices during your long fast you will be breathing in more prana life force energy that your body can use as fuel.

Can you Starve to Death from a Long Fast?

The answer is no. This is because when your fast continues to point where your body has no more non-vital tissue to break down to feed your vital organs, then your body will go into a great hunger. This is the signal the body uses to warn you that there is no more non-vital tissue left. At that point the long fast must be broken. At that point the body must have food again. However, that said, many break their long fast too early and deprive themselves of more optimal results and deeper cleansing and greater removal of all of the half dead senescent cells that cause some of the body's aging.

What is the Optimal Duration of a Long Fast?

Well, this, of course, depends upon many factors: how healthy you are to begin with, how much experience have you have with fasting, and what your goals are. But all things considered, I would say probably in the range of 60 days, which is 8 weeks, or two months for the non-expert. Of course, it is recommended that you read up on it, and if you have any contra symptoms don't be afraid to break your fast. Also, I would leave the longer long fasts, those over 60 days to the masters at this point.

The Long Fast – Living Several Hundred Years

Doing a yearly or bi-yearly long fast probably won't appeal to very many, but it is possible, and it does create the potential for a very long lifespan. And after you get past the fourth day you don't really feel hungry. This is hard to explain but it is true, you don't get hungry. Your body begins to feeds off of its fat reserves at first, and then after the fat reserves are used up, it begins to feed off of its non-vital tissues, so that your body's vital organs are always fed, and the results are that you don't feel hungry. After the 5th day you might feel somewhat nauseous but this will pass. After that you just need to keep on fasting. You really should read up on it first before you start. Shelton's fasting books are good, but there ae many others. You should also be aware of the contras that indicate that the fast should be broken. However, I have never had any of these contras. After about 20 days you will get somewhat weak. And it will be harder to speak because your mouth will get dry. And breaking the long fast is difficult and it is important to go slow. It takes two to three weeks after you break your long fast for your digestive system to adjust back to your normal eating routine.

The long fast is far and away the least expensive way to actually extend your life. After all, how much is it going to cost you to not eat anything for a month or more? But you must drink water. Water is needed for the ketone breakdown process. When you really get into fasting you will notice how people all around you and all over the world use food and drink as a tranquilizer. From my own personal experience, I think it is best to not talk about it to others, especially at your workplace, and especially if you are doing a long fast. My advice is to not talk about it at all at your work place. Most people will immediately think that it is too dangerous and that you should stop. They may even try to coerce you to stop. Many remember as a child being told that they must eat their food to stay strong and healthy. I have learned that it is best to not talk about my long fast (or any fast) at the work place when I am doing one. I just do my work and take part in the normal social conversations if I want to.

Some may say that doing a long fast is asking too much and it is too hard to do. But I say look at all the extra years it can give you. You can look at the long fast as spring cleaning. You can be happy for all of the senescent cells and toxins that are being removed. You can feel joy at knowing that you will live longer. I read an interesting article about a tree farm in England where trees were grown for producing long slender withy twigs and all of the branches at the tops were periodically cropped to harvest the withy twigs, and the interesting thing about this was the observation that these pruned and cropped tress lived far longer than the same trees that were not cropped and pruned. At least one comment on this phenomenon that I think might be correct was the observation that the pruned and cropped tress had their normal life cycle interrupted time after time, and they were reverted back to a more youthful part of their life cycle, time after time. The long fast of the immortal masters may have a similar affect.

A long fast may seem too difficult, but once you get started and get some momentum into it, it becomes easier because you sort of go on autopilot and it just becomes your new pattern and lifestyle and way of life. Many religions have yearly purification events and fasting is often a part of these events. Indeed, fasting is a purification practice and it is a purification practice for life extension. It should be added that fasting is not starving. It is true that your body's major organs: the heart, the lungs, the brain, the kidneys, and the liver have to be continually fed, and they are whether you are feeding or fasting. There are many fasting durations. Here is my list:

Short Fast	=	1-day to 1-week
Medium Fast	=	1-week to 1-month
Long Fast	=	1-month to 2-months

Although a 1-month long fast may sound daunting, it is doable. During any fast you will, of course, not eat any solid food, but again you must have water. Filtered water of course, and if you can afford it, lite water would be preferred. You can squeeze a little lime, lemon, or orange juice into your drinking water to help calm your stomach. During an intermediate or a long fast, you should plan on getting more sleep and you should avoid strenuous work. I do not exercise much after the 7th day of a fast. All fasts are valuable. The 1-day and 3-day fast will improve your digestion and elimination. A 1-week fast removes some of the stored fat and helps to eliminate excess weight. A 2-week fast begins to break down some of the nonessential tissues and gives your body a chance to eliminate some deeply buried toxins. All fasts are beneficial. All fasts contribute to body purification. And purification is key to life extension.

The serious life extension student should be open to allow adding fasting to their repertoire of life extension practices. Many people need others who are doing the same thing around them for support. But mastery means you can do it by yourself, on your own without needing the support of others to cheer you on. All of you reading this have the potential to become masters. I plan to continue doing my long fast at least once a year.

Most books, articles, and literature on fasting contain a disclaimer to protect the author by stating that they are not responsible in any way should any harm befall any person or persons from fasting. I also state that I cannot be held responsible in any way should any harm come any person or persons from fasting as a result of reading this book. I suggest that everyone interested in fasting for longevity and life extension should read up on it, and become familiar with any and all possible health concerns or contras that might result from fasting, and also if any health concern does occur, then the fast should be stopped. That said, I have never had negative health issues from the long fasts that I have done.

What Are the Most Important Things to Do to Go for 200 – 500 Years?

The items I list below are what I think are the most important things you should do to reach for the goal of living more than 200 Years.

Advanced Life Extension Practices

1. **Say your daily affirmations religiously and with powerful conviction**
When if they get stale, vary them, pick new ones from the lists

2. Become as toxin free as possible – in food, drink, thoughts, emotions
Incorporate advanced dietary choices - Lite Water

3. Advanced healing – orient your vacations towards healing
Hot springs
Radon health spas

3. Work on becoming the future human
Create daily life expectations of benevolence
Practice sending compassionate action
Develop your intuition to know the best choices
Daily move from "I" to 'WE" consciousness
Redefine bad-news into only a change is coming

4. Develop your interdimensional life extension connections
Learn shimmering
Learn soul fragmentation retrieval
Learn knowledge of the body's aura and kundalini and DNA
Learn telepathy
Learn bilocation and astral projection
Learn advanced manifestation

5. Rejuvenate using both internal practices and external technology
Lean advanced life extension energy exercises and meditations
Do a bi-yearly or yearly youthing visualization-meditation

6. Incorporate the secrets of the masters
Do a bi-yearly or yearly organ rejuvenation blue cocoon meditation
Do advanced breath work sessions
Do advanced fasting – work up to the long fast

7. Practice perfection daily
Perfection means mastery of the mind over the body
Perfection means evolving to ever higher levels of consciousness
Perfection means mastery of spiritual technology

Advanced Life Extension Affirmations

1. I say my daily affirmations for mastery of life extension and for creating a good day. I do this the first thing every day without fail and that is all there is to it!

2. I am a reality bender. I can bend reality such that the outcome is always good for me.

3. I affirm that as a life extender I intend to incorporate advanced breath work sessions.

4. I affirm that as a life extender I intend to incorporate advanced fasting practices.

5. I am learning to release all trauma and bad memories from this life and from all of my past lives, and I am learning to cultivate stillness. Indeed!

6. I am learning about the importance of the two-way communication of my personality complex to my soul and my soul's connection to its oversoul.

7. I am working on becoming the future human now by working with the future human exercises on a regular basis. Yes indeed, that is one of my goals!

8. I am incorporating the new revelations of the spiritual technologies of the cosmic egg, shimmering, though projection and telepathy. Oh yes!

9. I am a reality bender. I intend to bend my reality into the mastery of a life extender.

10. I, as a life extender, know that it is important to allow an on-going continuation of my life journey. I intend to focus on and allow an on-going continuation to unfold! Amen!

11. I, as a life extender know that continual healing of my major organs is needed and I do soul fragmentation retrieval and the thought-mind-power meditation to keep them healed and rejuvenated.

12. I am retrieving my lost soul fragments by requesting morning and evening cohabitation with my guides, the masters, and the angles, and by doing the soul fragment retrieval exercises. Yes!

13. I am open to utilizing technologies from the external science to further assist my life extension goals.

14. I know that greater life extension or a near immortality is linked to greater elimination of toxins, and I intend to gradually step up purifying my diet, my emotions and my thoughts.

15. I know that there will be many new antiaging and age reversal technologies coming in the near future and I will take advantage of the ones that are right for me.

16. I, as a life extender, know that there is a viral life extension movement going on right now and I intend to become a part of it and I expect to be carried along with the great life extension movement and greatly extend my own life. Indeed!

17. I, as a life extender, intend to do a yearly or bi-yearly Youthing Meditation Affirmation.

18. I, as a life extender, intend to the do a yearly or bi-yearly Thought-Mind-Power Blue Cocoon Rejuvenation Meditation.

19. I, as a life extender, will consider periodically adding the life extension practices of radon health mines and spas, and hot spring resorts.

20. I, as a life extender, will consider as my funds permit, adding lite water that has most of the heavy water removed because I know it can help heal and regenerate my body's tissues, organs, and structures.

21. I, as a life extender, know that my body is designed to last over 300 years and I'm going to go for an extended life span of _______ years that is right for me and that I feel comfortable about reaching. Oh, yes, I am!

22. I, as a life extender, am long past worrying about disease!

23. I, as a life extender, affirm that it is my intention to incorporate fasting and to continually work on letting it become a natural and easy life routine.

24. I, as a life extender, know that the long-fast is the cheapest way to go for life span of over 200 years, and I am going to consider doing the long-fast and I will be cognizant of the importance of going slowly and working into it by first doing many 1-day a week fasts, and then several 3-day a week fasts, and then a few 1-week fasts, and after that go for the longer fasts. I also will learn about and become familiar with all possible contras that could occur from a long fast.

25. I, as a life extender, know that breathwork mastery is the cheapest way to go for a life span of over 200 years, and am going to consider doing daily breathwork sessions of great power that can bring in vast amounts of extra energy with the inbreath and open chakras and can expel toxins and dead tissues of all kinds with the out breath, and I will add powerful visualization to add the prana and expel the toxins to my interdimensional body in my breathwork sessions.

26. I, as a life extender, intend to combine all of my life extension practices with breathwork mastery, fasting mastery and thought-mind-power mastery.

27. I, as a life extender, will work on allowing my sexuality and creativity to blossom into greater expression and fulfillment. Indeed!

What is totally absent from our culture is the notion that the legendary lifespans of the ancient immortals are not just legend – by using the long-fast, advanced breath-work, and perfecting advanced thought-mind power, it is an actual potential!

Closing Words and a Few Final Comments

I Challenge You to Go for It

Whatever lifespan you feel comfortable with, I challenge you to go for it. You can do it. Work with the practices, beginning-intermediate-advanced in this book. Say your daily affirmations, add exercise, yoga, meditation, etc. Do all of the visualization exercises and guided meditations. Alter your diet in food and drink for life extension. Get to your correct weight. Continually increase your life extension repertoire. Rotate your affirmations. Work with all of the speech-command body mastery exercises. Do the youthing and blue cocoon organ rejuvenation visualization-meditation. I challenge you to be better next year than you are now. I challenge you to actually do it and extend your life to become a mature person that always looks youthful and vital and healthy, and always has a powerful zest for life and always wants to learn more, and allows, to the best of their ability, the yumminess of life to seep in deeply. Whatever your current age is, I challenge you to pick an age you want to reach for and go for it. I challenge you to do it. You can do it, and that is all there is to it!

You can extend your life!

Reread the chapters you need to many times and begin to work on the topics discussed. Be more careful of your thoughts and your emotions and work on ensuring that they are of a higher consciousness.

By now you should realize that you can extend your life. I would like to see all of you do it. The first things you will need to do is to firmly decide that this is what you really want to do. And then get excited about it. Then you will need to start working with the life extension practices and I would suggest that it would be a good idea to make a daily, weekly, monthly and yearly plan or a schedule of the life extension protocols that you want to incorporate. And write in your schedule list the life extension practices and meditations and visualizations that you want to do to extend your life. And then do them!

Bibliography

Deng, MING-Dao, The Wandering Taoist, San Francisco: Harper & Row, !986

Michle, Gregor, Roxanne Cox, and Allan Watson, Pranayana the Breath of Yoga, Doubleview W.A.: Kalvalya Publications, 2012.

Orr, Leonard, Physical Immortality: The Science of Everlasting Life, Chico, CA: Inspiration Unoiversity, 1991.

Shelton, Herbert, Fast and Grow Young, Hygientic System VolIII, Dr Shelton's Health School, San Antonio, TX, 1934.

Shelton, Herbert, Fasting Can Save Your Life, National Hygiene Press, 1964-1981.

Vonderplanitz, Aajonus, We Want to Live: The Primal Diet, Santa Monica, CA: Carnelian Bay Castle Press, 1997.

Vonderplanitz, Aajonus, Recipe for Living without Disease, Santa Monica, CA: Carnelian Bay Castle Press, 1997.

Yogananda, Paramahansa, Autobiography of a Yogi, Self-Realization Fellowship, Los Angles, CA, 1946.

Age Reversal Slide Show, www.age-reversal.net

Life Extension Products, www.lifeextension.com

People Unlimited, www.peopleunlimitedinc.com

RAAD Fest, annual age reversal conference, www.raadfest.com

Sedona Journal of Emergence, www.Sedonajournal.com, articles revealing new life extension techniques, 1998 - 2020.

The Church of Perpetual Life, www.churchofperpetuallife.org

www.ingramcontent.com/pod-product-compliance
Lightning Source LLC
Chambersburg PA
CBHW051041250726
48656CB00001B/88